Leading Through Crisis

Intimate Stories of Teamwork, Caring, and Character in Graduate Medical Education

Edited by
Kathlyn E. Fletcher, MD, MA

Published by Ten16 Press, an imprint of Orange Hat Publishing, 2024
PB ISBN: 9781645387893
HC ISBN: 9781645387800

Copyrighted © 2024 by Kathlyn E. Fletcher
All Rights Reserved
Leading Through Crisis: Intimate Stories of Teamwork, Caring, and Character in Graduate Medical Education
Edited by Kathlyn E. Fletcher

Illustrations Copyrighted © 2024 by Lily Littrell

This publication and all contents within may not be reproduced or transmitted in any part or in its entirety without the written permission of the author.

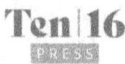

orangehatpublishing.com

For Jack, Lily, Jay, and Luke—
for understanding that I needed to do this
and adding laughter and perspective along the way.

For my fellow program directors—
for making this journey so much less lonely.

HOW TO USE THIS BOOK

While we would love for you to start with Chapter 1, familiarizing yourself with the conceptual framework first before delving into specific crisis topics, we expect many of you will first pick up this book in the heat of the moment and skip right to the most relevant chapter. Either way should work!

Our intent is that each chapter stands alone. When concepts apply to more than one chapter, we point you to chapters that contain additional information. For example, many chapters touch on the mental health and well-being of residents. Rather than being repetitive, we focus on the strategies that seem most applicable to the crisis at hand and refer to the other chapters with related information.

Each chapter is organized as follows:

1. Brief introduction to frame the crisis topic
2. Crisis story* told from the leader's point of view
3. Practical advice based on experience and/or the literature
4. Lessons learned: mistakes and things we could have done better
5. Summary table

*Unless otherwise noted, we have altered details and meshed stories together to protect the anonymity of the other people involved.

Enjoy!

KF

TABLE OF CONTENTS

Foreword
Beyond the Basics:
Preparing to Lead Residency Programs through Crises...13
    Holly J. Humphrey, MD, MACP

Preface..19
    Kathlyn E. Fletcher, MD, MA

Chapter 1
Leading Your Team Before, During, and After a Crisis:
A Conceptual Framework...23
    Mark A. Maltarich, PhD & Kathlyn E. Fletcher, MD, MA

Chapter 2
Practical Applications of the Conceptual Framework:
How to Lead Your Team Through a Crisis...44
    Mark A. Maltarich, PhD & Kathlyn E. Fletcher, MD, MA

Chapter 3
Leading Through a Mental Health Crisis of an Individual Resident..62
    Kathlyn E. Fletcher, MD, MA & Mara Pheister, MD

Chapter 4
Leading Through a Serious Illness and Death of a Resident..79
    Kathlyn E. Fletcher, MD, MA, Jillian Catalanotti, MD, MPH,
    & Amy S. Oxentenko, MD

Chapter 5
Leading Through a Crisis on Campus..98
    Matthew Goldblatt, MD & Kathlyn E. Fletcher, MD, MA

Chapter 6
Leading Through a Community Tragedy..110
    Mark Rasnake, MD, Glenn Paetow, MD, MACM,
    & Kathlyn E. Fletcher, MD, MA

Chapter 7
Leading Through a Pandemic...128
    Alec B. O'Connor, MD, MPH & Danielle S. Wallace, MD

Chapter 8
Leading During Times of Legal Uncertainty:
Legislative Disruption to Residency Training..147
    Amy Domeyer-Klenske, MD & Kate Dielentheis, MD

Chapter 9
Leading Through a Personal Crisis:
An Unexpected Serious Illness in the Program Director's Family...163
    Aimee K. Zaas, MD, MHS

Chapter 10
Taking Care of Yourself During a Crisis...175
    Mariah Quinn, MD, MPH, Mary Westergaard, MD,
    & Art Walaszek, MD

Chapter 11
Recovering from a Leadership Misstep..189
    David L. Hamel, Jr, MD, FACP

Chapter 12
What I Learned about Myself and My Team in My First Crisis as a Resident...................................197
    Rachel Goodman, MD

Finding Strength Together: Weathering a Natural Disaster with Colleagues....................................201
    Lawrence P.A. DeBellis, DO, MS

Navigating the Pandemic as a Resident and a Chief Resident..206
    Kaitlin Kyi, MD

Acknowledgments...209

CONTRIBUTORS

Jillian Catalanotti, MD, MPH
Department of Medicine
George Washington University School of Medicine and Health Sciences

Lawrence P.A. DeBellis, DO, MS
Department of Internal Medicine
Medical University of South Carolina

Kate Dielentheis, MD
Department of Obstetrics and Gynecology
Medical College of Wisconsin

Amy Domeyer-Klenske, MD
Department of Obstetrics and Gynecology
University of Wisconsin School of Medicine and Public Health

Kathlyn E. Fletcher, MD, MA
Department of Internal Medicine
Medical College of Wisconsin
Clement J. Zablocki VAMC

Matthew Goldblatt, MD
Department of Surgery
Medical College of Wisconsin

Rachel Goodman, MD
Department of Internal Medicine
Tufts University School of Medicine

David L. Hamel, Jr, MD, FACP
Department of Internal Medicine
Aurora Health Care

Holly J. Humphrey, MD, MACP
President, Josiah Macy Jr. Foundation

Kaitlin Kyi, MD
Department of Internal Medicine
University of Rochester School of Medicine and Dentistry

Mark A. Maltarich, PhD
Darla Moore School of Business, University of South Carolina

Alec B. O'Connor, MD, MPH
Department of Internal Medicine
University of Rochester School of Medicine and Dentistry

Amy S. Oxentenko, MD
Department of Internal Medicine
Mayo Clinic School of Medicine

Glenn Paetow, MD, MACM
Department of Emergency Medicine
Hennepin County Medical Center

Mara Pheister, MD
Department of Psychiatry and Behavioral Health
Medical College of Wisconsin

Mariah Quinn, MD, MPH
Department of Internal Medicine
University of Wisconsin School of Medicine and Public Health

Mark Rasnake, MD
Department of Internal Medicine
University of Central Florida College of Medicine

Danielle S. Wallace, MD
Department of Internal Medicine
University of Rochester School of Medicine and Dentistry

Art Walaszek, MD
Department of Psychiatry
University of Wisconsin School of Medicine and Public Health

Mary Westergaard, MD
Department of Emergency Medicine
University of Wisconsin School of Medicine and Public Health

Aimee K. Zaas, MD, MHS
Department of Internal Medicine
Duke University School of Medicine

FOREWARD
BEYOND THE BASICS: PREPARING TO LEAD RESIDENCY PROGRAMS THROUGH CRISES

by Holly J. Humphrey, MD, MACP

President, Josiah Macy Jr. Foundation

I wish that this book—essentially a how-to manual for managing crises in residency programs—had existed in 1987 when I was chief medical resident at The University of Chicago Medical Center. I would have read it cover to cover and kept it on hand as a quick reference guide. And, when I became director of the internal medicine residency program in 1989, I would have read it again and continued to use it as a resource. I say this because, back then, as a pulmonologist, I felt very well prepared to manage patients and their medical crises. As chief resident and then as a new program director, however, I had much less experience managing colleagues and assisting them with work-related challenges, particularly during moments of crisis when it is crucial "to get it right."

I would have found the very practical contents of this book helpful in each of my leadership roles at the University of Chicago—even after I became dean for medical education. The first chapter lays out an evidence-based framework to guide leadership team functioning before, during, and after a crisis. Subsequent chapters walk readers through different types of crises that may occur in a local community (e.g., a natural disaster), on an academic health center campus (e.g., a fatal shooting), within a residency program (e.g., the serious illness or death of a resident)—or even in all these settings at once (e.g., a pandemic). It also includes a chapter on taking care of yourself while managing a crisis.

Fortunately, during my time as a residency program director, whether I had a serious crisis or a simple query, I had three vitally important resources to lean on for guidance. One was my mentor, who was also the chair of medicine, Dr. Arthur Rubenstein. He was so superbly skilled as a mentor (he's retired now) that an annual faculty mentorship award at the University of Chicago is named in his honor. My other resource was the Association of Program Directors in Internal Medicine (APDIM), which enabled me to build close connections with experienced colleagues, some of whom had been program directors for decades, as well as peers, who had become program directors around the same time as me. I attended APDIM's meetings religiously, every spring and fall, for years. I even served as president of the organization for a year and co-authored the first edition of its *Chief Resident's Manual*, which—now in its 25th edition—is currently titled *A Textbook for Today's Chief Medical Resident*. The third resource was the residents and chief residents in our program. They were the day-to-day experts on what was working and what needed improvement. Essentially, Dr. Rubenstein, my APDIM community, and the residents and chief residents taught me how to be a residency program director, including advising me through management of crises big and small.

In fact, Dr. Rubenstein played a critical role in managing the impact of two simultaneous crises on my co-workers and the residents in our program. On a late summer day in 1996, I learned that a member of my own family had died. A few hours later, while preparing to take time off to be with my family, I was informed that one of our residents had not reported to work and was missing. Sadly, that night, after holding on to hope all day, we learned that the resident had died. It was the most personally and professionally challenging day of my entire fourteen-year tenure as program director.

For some time afterward, things carried on, but felt upside down—everywhere I turned, while holding space for my own grief, there were other grievers to console, work to do, and patients to care for. I had never experienced anything like the emotional turmoil and mental demands of that time—nor have I since. While I left Chicago to help my family deal with our private loss, Dr. Rubenstein abandoned his vacation and immediately returned to the city to manage the loss within our work family. It felt like a gift having him step into the work crises on my behalf; not only could I focus on my family situation, but I knew my residency program colleagues and our residents—including then first-year resident Dr. Kathlyn Fletcher, now the editor and lead author of this book—were in the hands of a singular leader who freely shared his wisdom and compassion.

Dr. Rubenstein shared his own emotions freely and encouraged everyone else in the program to do the same. He explained that they should focus their energy on comforting the family of the resident who had died, without worrying about saying the wrong thing. The only wrong thing, according to him, was to say nothing at all. When I returned to work, it was to a team of colleagues and residents who said they felt listened to and cared for in my absence, and I was profoundly grateful.

Sometime later, I realized that as terrible as the whole of that experience was, I had learned a tremendous amount about the importance of empathy, compassion, and trust in the workplace—about the need for team members to look out for each other and support each other. I added those lessons to the many others I had picked up along the way.

By 2003, when I left the residency program to become dean for medical education, I had begun developing a handful of practices and principles that, eventually, my leadership team and I came to rely on as we managed the medical education enterprise. It is only now, however, that I recognize those practices and principles as a cohesive set of leadership tools because, during my tenure as dean, they each evolved separately and informally, always subject to adaptations and revisions as needed.

My leadership team and I frequently communicated about these practices and principles to staff—through speeches, meetings, and reviews—and, later, we would sometimes see our words around the office, written on sticky notes and stuck to computers, desks, phones, and bulletin boards. We used these informal practices and principles very intentionally to establish a tone of mutual respect in the office and give everyone, regardless of their role, guidelines for handling various situations. Below, the practices and principles are presented together for the first time as a cohesive set with explanatory text.

1. **De-escalate.** This was our most well-established practice. Hospitals are extremely emotionally charged environments. We frequently had students, residents, and faculty turning up in the program director's office (and later the dean's office) in heightened states of anger, anxiety, frustration, etc., because something had gone wrong and a patient was almost or actually harmed. My mantra with the program office staff (and later the dean's office staff) was that our job was to defuse emotion and to communicate a sense of calm because only in this frame of mind would we find a way to understand and resolve the issue.

2. **Take the high road.** In addition to de-escalation, when someone was upset and demanding action, we always steered those involved toward the high road. We asked them to remember that everyone was on the same team and working toward the same goal of high-quality patient care. We would ask them for their side of the story and for enough time to gather information from the others involved, reminding them that, together, we would make things better. We also asked them to look at the data and think the very best of people that the data would support.

3. **Ask "What can we learn from this?"** In the middle of difficult circumstances, we always asked, "Do we have all of the necessary information, or are we missing certain perspectives or data points for resolution?" After resolution, in the spirit of nurturing growth mindsets and self-reflection among those involved, we talked about what could be learned from the situation—whether it was something that an individual(s) could do differently, a situation that could be avoided in the future, or a gap in the system that leadership needed to remedy.

4. **Always express gratitude.** Depending on the situation, there is usually someone who has helped or tried to help, and it is always worth seeking them out and saying thank you. This is an easy, powerful, and often-overlooked secret to success.

5. **Act on behalf of the most vulnerable and you're probably doing the right thing.** In any conflict or crisis situation, there often are power imbalances between the people involved. When a faculty member and a resident find themselves in a disagreement, for example, the faculty member usually, but not always, occupies the more powerful position, while the resident, having less agency and authority, is in a less powerful position. In such situations, the person(s) in the more advantageous position should recognize their position of power and act on behalf of those who are in the vulnerable position.

These practices and principles are not specifically about crisis management, but I believe they can and should be applied in all situations where clear, committed, and compassionate leadership is required, particularly during a crisis or when working to avert one. As I read this book, I noticed that some of these same or similar principles—expressed differently—were applied to many different types of crisis situations. However, while my practices and principles are based on my own experiences and were developed in reaction to situations that occurred fairly regularly, the book is intended to help you be proactive, and its guidance is based on a thorough review of the literature, both from business and psychology. Through their reviews, the authors have identified ways to optimize leadership team function before, during, and after a crisis. Their evidence-based advice is far more extensive, thorough, and specific than my more general practices and principles.

I believe that those of us who take on the responsibility for training the next generation of physicians have a fundamental obligation to continually improve the experiences of our residents. Residency is a very vulnerable time in the professional and personal development of physicians, and when they are under our watch, we owe them our absolute best. As Dr. Francis Peabody famously once said about patients, but I like to change up just a little to remind myself that it applies equally well to residents: *The secret to the care of the resident is in caring for the resident.*[1]

---

[1]   Peabody FW. The Care of the Patient. JAMA 1927; 88(12):877-882.

To that end, my hope is that all chief residents and residency program directors have a trusted mentor like Dr. Rubenstein to turn to when needed. I also hope that all program directors find their professional association, whether it be the APDIM or a similar organization for program directors in other specialties, to be a powerful resource where they can connect with peers and access useful programming and helpful informational materials.

Regardless of these hopes, my advice to you—whether you are a residency program director, assistant director, coordinator, chief resident, or serve in a related role—is to read this book and learn from the experiences and expertise of those who are engaged in the same work that you are privileged to do. Read it in its entirety, share and discuss it with others on your team, and keep it close at hand. It is a practical resource that will help you manage all sorts of challenges, big and small, while also preparing you and your teammates to respond with compassion and grace when difficult days come.

PREFACE

December 13, 2021, Wisconsin. It is 6:00 a.m. and 39 degrees. I am running toward the bluff at Klode Park with one of my stalwart workout friends, Cassie. We have been exercising outdoors since the COVID-19 shutdown in March 2020. During our run, she helps me keep going as we compare notes about life and work. We're both thinking about writing a book, but on different topics. This morning, as we start down the bluff in the dark, I finally understand "why" I need to write this book: Some of the most challenging parts of leading a residency program through the darkness of a crisis—or leading any program, for that matter—would be easier if someone who has "been there" can help guide you. It's like having a stalwart workout friend who stays by your side when you're barely able to breathe, let alone participate in a conversation. We curve to the east, and Lake Michigan, framed by a glowing orange and pink sky, is before us as we run side by side. These are the moments that make frigid early-morning workouts worthwhile.

Indeed, we are not alone with our challenges. Simply knowing others are with you in moments of darkness is powerful. The culture of the past, where leaders were made to feel they needed to face things alone, is gradually shifting to a healthier work environment. And not a moment too soon. This book is intended to ensure that, even when facing a novel challenge, you can benefit from the lived experiences of others. You most definitely do not have to walk alone.

The COVID-19 years have provided us all with myriad leadership crises. They have shown us there are nuances in leading graduate medical education that deserve attention. While we will cover COVID-19 and other natural disasters in this book, the last four years have challenged our leadership in many realms besides those related to caring for patients under conditions of great uncertainty. For example, the pandemic itself exacerbated mental health problems in faculty and residents. Those years also brought tumultuous events sparked by the death of George Floyd and the subsequent Black Lives Matter protests of 2020. Then there was the overturning of Roe v. Wade in 2022. We continued to see other community tragedies such as the Fourth of July shooting in Highland Park, IL, and the school shooting in Uvalde, TX. Anti-Semitism, Islamophobia, hatred aimed at any group, and conflicts across the globe affect us as leaders and individual residents whose identities and families are impacted. Facing these events and their consequences demanded much from leaders.

Once we find ourselves in a crisis, character comes into play. I have come to understand that leading through a crisis requires courage, honesty, perspective, and love. You may think a crisis just happens; that we don't choose to take on a crisis. I disagree. Some people do walk away from leadership positions as a crisis unfolds. By staying, we choose to lead. Knowing the character strengths that help us lead effectively through a crisis is essential. Explicitly calling our strengths to mind in difficult times helps us recognize and counter the emotions that hold us back from acting. As Brené Brown points out in *Atlas of the Heart*, anxiety and fear are powerful emotions. They are also normal emotions. However, anxiety leads to worry and/or avoidance—neither of which are particularly helpful in a crisis. Understanding what causes anxiety and fear in ourselves is a first step toward garnering the courage to move forward.

Road map to the book
Because much of our work occurs within leadership teams, our book begins with two chapters introducing a conceptual framework grounded in the organizational psychology and business literature on leading teams. You will see concepts within this framework that you already know implicitly, such as build trust within your team. These concepts are intuitive but not obvious. Frameworks can be helpful because they make instinctive actions explicit. Frameworks are informed by the research evidence and therefore inform evidence-based strategies and support consistent decision-making and leadership. At the time of a crisis, you may be able to add people with certain skillsets to your team or physical resources (except personal protective equipment!) in a timely way. However, it's too late to add trust; trust must be built over time. So, explicit efforts to build trust matter before a crisis happens. The framework reminds us how and what to prepare ahead.

Because we can't anticipate and address every specific situation that you will face as a program director, we organized the next seven chapters around representative types of crises from which you can extrapolate. We deliberately sought a range of voices from across the United States—including residents—to offer readers a comprehensive perspective. We share mistakes we made along the way in the hope you will be able to avoid them. We highlight the importance of the humility and honesty required of leaders. We also include chapters about taking care of yourself during a crisis and recovering from leadership mistakes. The last chapter is comprised of reflections provided by residents or chief residents to help us understand what crises look like from their viewpoints.

Conclusion

No book can prepare you for the hardest days you will have as program director. You may have to pick up the pieces after a hurricane or a mass shooting in your community. You may face local or national political strife or unrest. You will likely have individual residents who will tell you scary, heavy things that require you to bear witness and then guide them to safety. You and your team will have to lead through these situations, absorbing the losses that define the crises and grieving as you lead. You will see that many leadership principles described are relevant across the varied crises you will face. Adjust the advice to your specific situations and your own personal style. My hope is that by sharing generalizable advice, collective wisdom, and the available research, we give you a place to start when the next crisis begins.

I dread getting out of bed for December workouts. What keeps me going? 1) Knowing I do not have to design the workout myself, 2) having friends at the park who will run beside me and not judge me when I can't run and talk at the same time, and 3) realizing that for a few short minutes before sunrise, when the sky is the color of fire, I am part of something bigger.

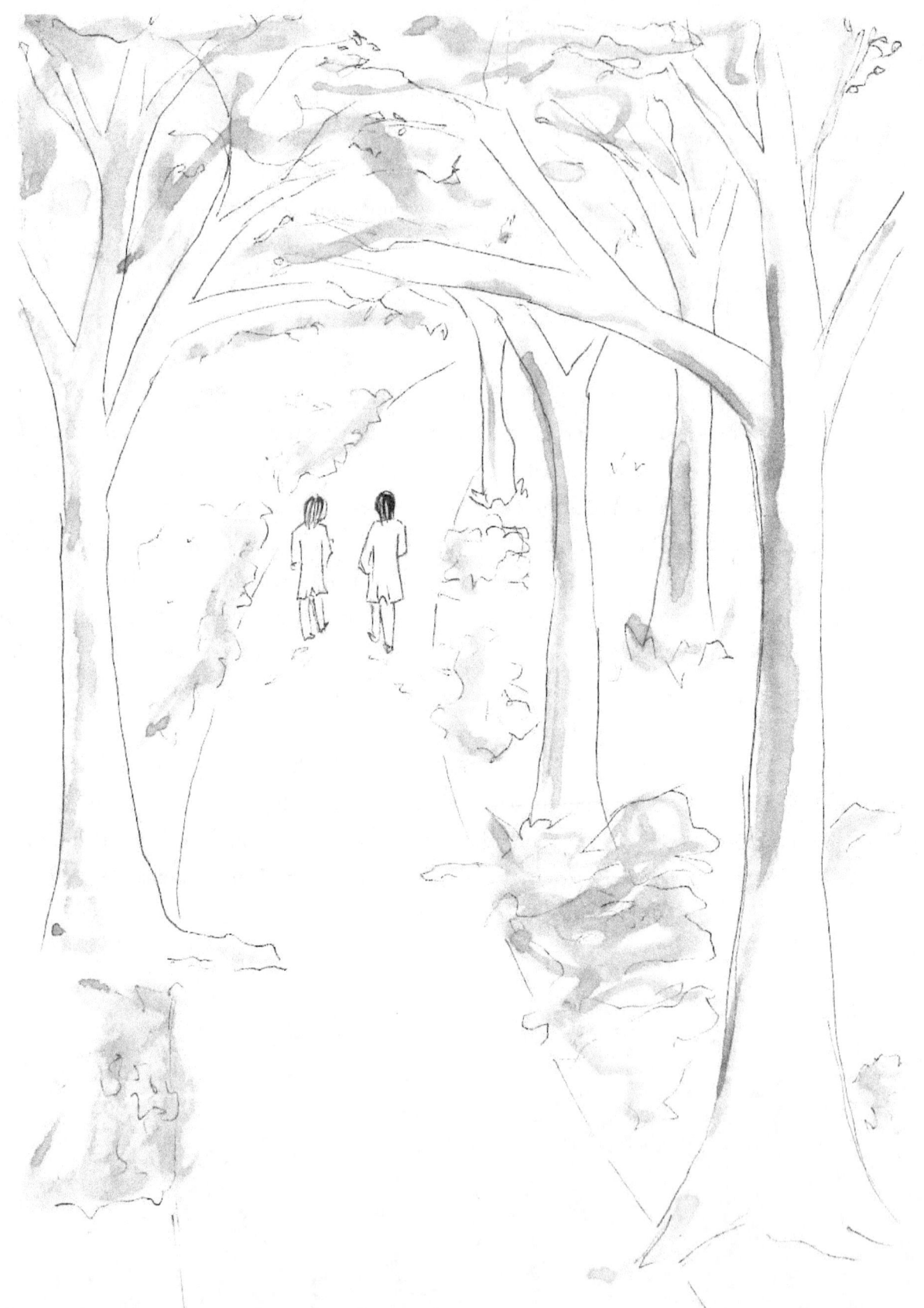

CHAPTER 1

Leading Your Team Before, During, and After a Crisis: A Conceptual Framework

Mark A. Maltarich, PhD

Darla Moore School of Business, University of South Carolina

Kathlyn E. Fletcher, MD, MA

Medical College of Wisconsin

Chapter 1 is for nerds like us who love conceptual frameworks. We synthesize important ideas and relevant literature from the social sciences into a framework of team functioning during crisis. This framework suggests how to best approach the daily work of directing a residency program, illustrated by examples and practical advice from our own experiences.

A story about lack of teamwork
My (KF's) residency program had a problem. It was early in my tenure, and more than 10% of our residents reported at least one duty hour violation during a routine monitoring period. The Accreditation Council for Graduate Medical Education (ACGME) rule most often broken by my residents stipulates that they are not allowed to work more than 80 hours a week, averaged over four weeks. I met with every resident who had reported a violation to understand the root causes. Within a few months, the ACGME imposed a formal citation on our program for not adhering to the duty hour rules.

I didn't ask for input from my associate program directors (APDs) before implementing a solution. Why? I was new in my leadership position. Some APDs didn't trust me yet, and one routinely and acrimoniously disagreed with me in meetings while others sat silent. When discussing how to address the duty hour violations and the ACGME citation, no one offered their own ideas. My solution to our problem, a day float system, was effective but despised (to this day) by the residents. It took four years of additional improvements and communication with the ACGME to have the citation removed from our program.

Working in teams is complex. Each teammate has unique needs, preferences, personality traits, strengths, vulnerabilities, and goals. Any two teammates have a unique relationship, including their experiences with, knowledge about, and attitudes toward each other. The complexity of relationships increases with each new teammate, and the difficulty of managing the team expands accordingly.

Managing all the tasks and relationships on a team is daunting under the best of circumstances, but in a crisis, it can become overwhelming. Graduate Medical Education (GME) leaders, while experienced in thinking systematically about patient care and the education of trainees, may be novices when it comes to leading large teams through an emergency. The good news, though, is that social science can help. A large body of research on teams offers GME leaders a road map for managing teams during crisis.

THE SCIENTIFIC BASIS FOR TEAMWORK

Researchers in social psychology, industrial/organizational psychology, sociology, behavioral economics, and organizational behavior have been studying teams for almost a century (Roethlisberger & Dickson, 1939), especially in the last three decades (Mathieu et al., 2017; Salas et al., 2008). Early work focused on predicting outcomes based on teammate and task characteristics. For example, Tziner and Eden (1985) studied two-man military tank crews, finding that specific combinations of soldiers with high (or low) ability and high (or low) motivation resulted in performance that could substantially exceed or fall short of what would be expected, based on the pair's average level of ability and motivation. Steiner (1972) attributed these differences to problems of coordination and teamwork. Coordination and teamwork work in concert with task characteristics (such as work interdependence) and team configurations (such as diversity of ability) to make the most of teams and drive performance.

More recently, researchers have studied team interactions and processes in laboratory or classroom settings (Ellis et al., 2003; Homan, 2007; Maltarich et al., 2018) and in workplace settings (Stewart et al., 2012), including medical environments (Hughes et al., 2016; Yun et al., 2005). They have studied the role of teams' experience working together (Wolfson & Mathieu, 2018) and teams of experts that have not worked together previously (Salas et al., 2006). Especially relevant to our purpose are studies of team adaptation in the face of change (Baard et al., 2014; LePine, 2003, 2005; Maynard et al., 2015) and teamwork in extreme environments or crisis (Driskell, 2018; Stachowski et al., 2009).

As an example of the complex processes studied by researchers, Wolfson and Mathieu (2021) examined task specialization and social relations as predictors of performance among cycling teams in the Union Cycliste Internationale World Tour. They found that the talent of cycling teams' members explained less than 10% of the variance in teams' performance. More important were 1) the selection of riders with race-appropriate specializations (e.g., sprint, mountain climbing) and 2) the experience riders had working together ("shared team task-specific experience," or STTE). Teams of riders that were well-suited for a race performed better *only* when they had shared experience. Teamwork considerations became even more important when conditions were extreme:

> *"During downhill sprints riders go upwards of 122 km per hour (Clarke, 2015), and must stay extremely close to one another to gain aerodynamic advantages (Martin et al., 2007). In these instances, miscoordination of even a few centimeters, could literally mean the difference between victory and a potentially life-threatening crash. Even on flat surfaces, teammates orchestrate a finely tuned sequence of rotating the lead rider to maximize overall team speed while minimally taxing featured riders . . . when the situation is extreme, the relevant competencies are high, and so is the STTE, the full benefits of [team capabilities] and [their social ties] are realized."*
> *(Wolfson & Mathieu, 2018)*

In the following section, we synthesized high-quality teams research to develop a concrete conceptual framework to help GME leaders prepare for and lead through the kinds of crises they will inevitably face. Before we get into the details, though, two overarching principles deserve special mention—the concept of foundation work, and the need to manage both taskwork and teamwork.

Foundation work

Foundation work is the effort a team exerts to develop a shared understanding of their core values, the work and working environment, team conditions such as trust and cohesion, and decisions about how conflict will be managed. Early foundational experiences can have lasting effects (Meister et al., 2020). For example, Mathieu and Rapp (2009) studied thirty-two teams of MBA students operating simulated firms over a semester. Early on, teams completed a team charter which identified individual strengths and weaknesses, discussed team member work styles and schedule preferences, and recorded negotiated procedures for coordination and conflict resolution. At the same time, teams developed strategies, set performance targets, and decided on systems to monitor success and adapt as necessary. The best-performing teams had a combination of well-formed charters and sound strategies at the onset. Group norms established during chartering help teams adapt to unexpected disruptions (Sverdrup et al., 2017). These effects stem from the chartering itself, not simply from team bonding or cohesiveness (Courtright et al., 2017). In KF's story, she spent little time developing foundational relationships and finding common ground with her team. She simply took over from the previous (and beloved) program director, who had made most crisis decisions on his own.

Taskwork and teamwork

A common feature of the crises described in this book is that the potential fallout is not simply operational (the hated day float solution) and technical (having an ACGME citation for four years). It is human (KF's team was not invested in the solution). This means leaders and teams must pay attention to the task at hand, but also cannot lose sight of teammate attitudes and behaviors directed toward each other. A central lesson from the teams research is that *taskwork*—the assignment of duties, coordination of activity, monitoring, and feedback—must be balanced with the *teamwork* aspects of leadership: motivation, emotion, belonging, trust, and meaningful work (Crawford & LePine, 2013; Driskell et al., 2018; Marks et al., 2001). Managing taskwork and managing teamwork are related, but distinct, leadership functions (Fisher, 2014). Teamwork planning promotes positive team processes such as openness and trust, which were clearly missing in the early part of KF's tenure as PD.

Summary and more good news

Teams science provides specific guidance for GME programs weathering a crisis by directing attention to the most impactful elements of team structure and function. In the next section, we describe a framework which anchors the theoretical and empirical research in real-world examples.

THE FRAMEWORK

Figure 1 synthesizes more than half a century of research into a single model. It is tailored to provide a concrete, actionable, and phased framework for team leadership in the context of graduate medical education programs.

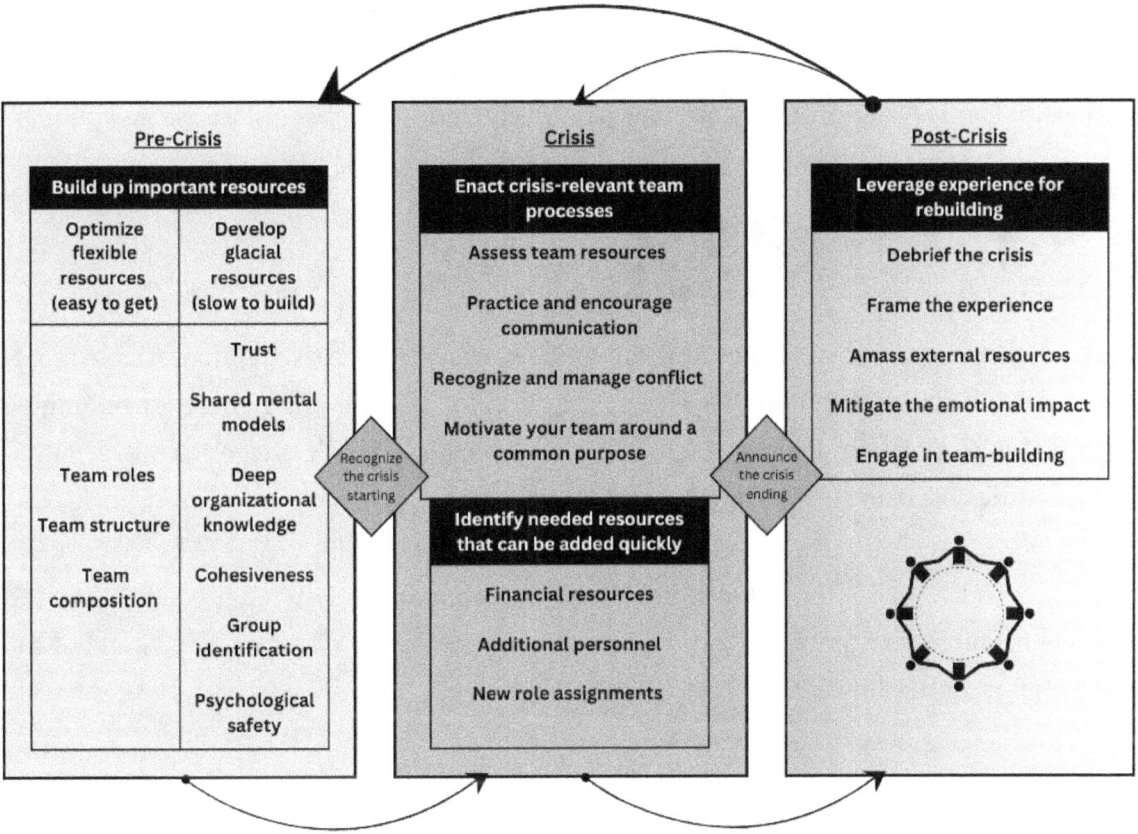

Figure 1: Actions to create high-performing teams before, during, and after a crisis

Overview

The figure is divided into distinct phases—pre-crisis, crisis, and post-crisis—consistent with the idea that each phase requires different leadership approaches (Marks et al., 2001). Ideally, the pre-crisis phase is the time to do foundational team-building work. The crisis phase, likely chaotic, is when a team is required to make quick adjustments. Flexibility and adaptability reign during the crisis phase when decision-making is hampered by time constraints, rapid change, information shortages, and stress. The post-crisis phase allows for reflection and recovery and the emergence of a "new normal."

The distinctions between phases are clear in the figure, but they can be fuzzy in practice. Recognizing the transitions, communicating them, and moving the team from one stage to the next are all vital to effective crisis management. Kent & Granqvist (2020) studied this in storm chasing teams, where group leaders combined explicit statements and symbolic changes (e.g., turning the chase vehicle's hazard lights on) to clearly signal to the whole team they had entered the "chase mode." This clear communication ensured that team members uniformly perceived and adjusted to the phase change, adjusting their behavior quickly and in unison. In medical education, discussing an evolving crisis in explicit language with your leadership team ("The spread of coronavirus is likely to impact us soon; we are now preparing") could be the equivalent of the storm chasers' flipping on the hazard lights.

The Pre-Crisis Phase

Leaders must prepare for crises even if the specifics of a given crisis are unknowable in advance. The challenge then becomes leveraging the calm of a pre-crisis phase for building a team that is adaptable and resilient across a range of challenges. We categorize the resources needed as flexible (can change quickly) and glacial (change slowly).

Optimize Flexible Resources

Flexible resources are those that can be adjusted without delay when needed. Some of the most important flexible resources are described below.

Team roles

Team roles can be formal or informal. While taskwork is often attached to formal titles, such as APD for Wellness or Patient Safety Chief Resident, it can also be informally distributed to others. In the TREO model (Mathieu, Tannenbaum et al., 2015), team roles include 1) *organizer*, who structures work, coordinates, and monitors progress toward goals; 2) *doer*, who focuses on task execution; 3) *challenger*, who plays devil's advocate or questions assumptions; 4) *innovator*, who introduces creative solutions; 5) *team builder*, who promotes unity and mutual support among team members, and 6) *connector*, who spans team boundaries to interface with outside stakeholders. In medical education teams, the program coordinator, administrators, chief residents, APDs, PD, and core faculty likely take on these roles.

In the pre-crisis phase, these roles might be informal and fluid. Several team members may offer innovative ideas or challenge assumptions. In a crisis, everyone becomes more of a doer. During the COVID-19 pandemic, for example, APDs and core faculty members took on substantially more clinical work, which left a vacuum in other roles such as providing formal education, building rapport, and organizing programs. As the crisis unfolded and some administrative professionals were furloughed, program coordinators took on more work, which left them with less bandwidth for the connector role they often played. Under these rapidly evolving circumstances, leaders need to be more explicit in assigning specific roles to ensure that nothing falls through the cracks. Time spent identifying and developing certain teammates for these roles during the pre-crisis phase may pay off when a crisis occurs.

Team structure

Team structure denotes the distribution of responsibility and authority. Teams can be arranged hierarchically, with decision-making and coordination centralized in the PD, or teams can be fully decentralized, with individual members given a lot of decision-making latitude. Research indicates that different structures help teams respond to different types of stress. Matching the structure to the work can help teams face stressful situations effectively (Drach-Zahavy & Freund, 2007).

In GME programs with multiple training sites, cultivating a decentralized structure may be especially important. Site APDs may be better equipped to interface with the local institutional leadership to represent the needs, capacity, and capability of the residency. During the initial COVID-19 surge, KF's program had to consider involvement in surge plans at the VA hospital and the main hospital. The VA site director was instrumental in proposing the most realistic and least disruptive contributions of the residents with the fewest unintended negative consequences.

Team composition

PDs who have tried to get approval for new personnel budget lines might have salient experiences with bureaucratic resistance, but human capital resources can potentially be added quickly. When elective surgeries shut down early in the pandemic, anesthesia residents and faculty at some hospitals were redeployed from the operating rooms to the ICUs to help meet the increased critical care demands. A crisis often compels institutions to consider unprecedented, uncharacteristic creativity and flexibility with respect to personnel.

Develop Glacial Resources

Glacial resources can only be changed over time through investment in relationships and team-building. Glacial resources are what make the pre-crisis phase so important to crisis management—by the time you need glacial resources, it's too late to do much about them. You can build on pre-existing team strengths to build important glacial resources (Table 1).

Team trust

Researchers define trust as *a willingness to be vulnerable to another based on a perception of the other's ability, benevolence, integrity, and predictability* (Mayer et al., 1995; Mishra, 1996). Trust is complex because it can be between two individuals, but it can also exist among subgroups or between the leader and the team. It can be reciprocal or asymmetric: I trust you, but you don't trust me (Korsgaard et al., 2015). Trust within teams builds over time, shaped by individuals' propensity to trust others, leadership style, shared experience over time, the nature of team interactions, and specific trust-building exercises (Han & Harms, 2010; Jarvenpaa et al., 1998; Salas et al., 2006). If KF had asked her team for help with the ACGME duty hour citation, she might have earned their trust sooner. If the APDs had trusted her, they might have proposed more robust "outside the box" solutions rather than the "Band-Aid" she designed.

Shared mental models

Shared mental models (SMMs) are sets of knowledge about the task and environment that help teammates interpret, understand, explain, and predict task-relevant phenomena (Mathieu et al., 2000; Rouse & Morris, 1986). Teams benefit from shared mental models—especially of their environmental conditions and others' actions, the drivers of success, and the potential consequences of decisions (DeChurch & Mesmer-Magnus, 2010). Shared mental models can be especially impactful in complex teams of experts (Cannon-Bowers, 1993) such as healthcare teams (McComb & Simpson, 2014).

Deep organizational knowledge

Also known as transactive memory systems (Brandon & Hollingshead, 2004; Peltokorpi, 2008), deep organizational knowledge provides shared understanding of what each person knows, what they do, and what they need to accomplish in their work. This knowledge develops over time and with shared experience, shaped by team inputs (such as technical competence), task elements (such as interdependence of the work and rewards), and stress (see Ren & Argote for an excellent review) (Ren & Argote, 2011).

Cohesiveness

Shared commitment to the task and to liking each other as teammates (Hausknecht et al., 2009) drives group cohesiveness, process, and performance (Gross & Martin, 1952). Leadership style—especially transformational leadership (Bass, 1999; Jung & Sosik, 2002)—helps build cohesiveness, as does similarity in demographics and values among teammates (Olie et al., 2020; Seong et al., 2015). Like other glacial resources, cohesiveness develops over time as a function of shared experience and successes (Acton et al., 2020; Mathieu, Kukenberger, et al., 2015). Indeed, highly functioning teams often start meetings by highlighting recent successes of those in the group to help build cohesiveness.

Group identification

Leaders influence group identification by promoting a common identity and the idea that team members rely on each other for their joint success (Fisher & Wakefield, 1998; Henry et al., 1999; Hogg et al., 2007; Miller et al., 2020). Research highlights that demographic similarity facilitates the development of group identification, but less visible aspects of diversity also matter a lot for how members come to identify with their group (van Knippenberg et al., 2007). The process of building a group identity is complex and often requires intentional effort.

Psychological safety

Psychological safety is defined as the extent to which the team setting promotes open discussion, speaking up, and seeking feedback (Edmondson, 1999). Psychological safety has been studied extensively in workplace decision-making teams (Edmondson & Lei, 2014; Frazier et al., 2017; Newman et al., 2017). Supportive leadership is a key antecedent of psychological safety (Bienefeld & Grote, 2014), and collective accountability for outcomes helps teammates make the most of it (O'Neill, 2009).

Pre-Crisis Phase Conclusions

Built on the principles of foundation work and balancing taskwork with teamwork, our framework takes a view of the pre-crisis phase as an opportunity to gradually build valuable team resources. Some resources accumulate more quickly and others very gradually. Good leadership in the pre-crisis phase requires anticipating and planning for possible crises. It requires building a team with the capacity for coordinated and effective adaptation during crisis.

The Crisis Phase

Distinguishing between flexible and glacial resources becomes especially important in a crisis. Leaders must assess the situation and determine what resources are available and which to deploy. Here, we describe the key team processes in a crisis, which team resources matter to them, and why.

Assess Team Resources

Consider the team resources described in the pre-crisis phase. Once you enter the crisis phase, take stock of those resources and identify deficits. Chapter 2 has suggestions for how to measure these resources. Try to obtain the flexible resources you need. You may need to work around deficits in glacial resources (see Chapter 2 for suggestions).

Table 1: Glacial resources, existing team strengths, and interventions to strengthen the resources		
Team resources	**Existing team strengths**	**Interventions to strengthen resources**
Team trust	• Individual differences • Shared experience • Similarities	• Participative leadership • Team-building exercises • Accentuate similarities
Shared mental models	• Similarity in training/background • Shared experience • Time	• Clear communication • Scenario planning • After-action reviews • Collective rewards/recognition
Deep organizational knowledge	• Distributed expertise • Team familiarity/trust • Interdependence	• Explicit sharing of expertise • Group training • Inclusive planning/strategizing

Cohesiveness	• Leadership style • Demographic and value similarity • Shared success	• Transformational leadership • Accentuate similarities • Highlight success • Collective rewards/recognition
Group identification	• Previously shared experiences • Similarities and differences in experience, demographics, and viewpoint	• Team identification of common values • Highlight successes dependent on multiple team members • Call out the importance of diversity in viewpoints
Psychological safety	• Supportive leadership • Reward interdependence	• Individual consideration • Active listening • Collective rewards/recognition

Questions for leaders at the start of a crisis:

- What team resources (e.g., trust, shared mental models) do we have, and which do we lack?
- Which resources will we need for meeting this challenge?
- Which adjustments can be made in response to a crisis, and which cannot?
- What team strategies will help us leverage our strengths and offset our weaknesses?

Practice and Encourage Communication

Communication is required for effective teamwork (Ilgen et al., 2005; Mesmer-Magnus & DeChurch, 2009). Frequent, high-quality information sharing within a team promotes performance (Marlow et al., 2018). Teams lacking shared mental models and deep organizational knowledge are likely to have inefficient, haphazard exchanges of low-quality information and a low ratio of information offered to information requested (Entin & Serfaty, 1999; Sexton et al., 2018), even in healthcare crises (Stachowski et al., 2009).

A crisis may require a team to develop new communication processes because valued information may be scarce or come in an overwhelming flood. For instance, in an evolving natural disaster (Chapter 6), weather predictions, local evacuation plans, and facility-specific plans can lead to confusing and conflicting information. Early in the COVID-19 pandemic (Chapter 7), some residency leadership groups used frequent team huddles to make sense of and share the vast amount of incoming information.

Recognize and Manage Conflict

Good processes for assessing and addressing conflict and conflict management are necessary in crisis because some decisions must be made quickly based on limited information. Conflict can take several forms: *task conflict, relationship conflict,* and *process conflict.* As the labels imply, task conflict involves differing opinions around the nature of the task and strategies to pursue; relationship conflict involves person-centered adversity around values and personality clashes; process conflict denotes friction around how teams will operate and make decisions. The consensus is that task conflict and process conflict can be productive and promote good decision-making. Relationship conflict, in contrast, hinders performance while causing dissatisfaction with the team and the task (de Wit et al., 2012; Jehn & Mannix, 2001). Relationship conflict should be resolved rapidly during a crisis. High-performing teams have conflict effectively around ideas but avoid interpersonal friction.

Glacial team resources affect conflict in two ways. First, congruent values and priorities provide an objective basis for sorting through and evaluating different perspectives and proposals and smoothing the conflict management process. Second, team trust, cohesion, and goal congruity reflected in shared mental models allow a team to interpret ambiguous tense interactions generously—categorizing them as well-intentioned task conflict rather than as relationship conflict (e.g., the sharp tone of voice on a phone call interpreted as stress of the speaker instead of anger at the listener), though this area is under-investigated.

A Graduate School Story to Illustrate Conflict

As a first-semester PhD student, I (MM) attended a research presentation where junior faculty presented work in progress to senior faculty. The presenter had gotten as far as the title slide when the venerated old man of the department raised his hand. "Charlie," he said with mischief in his eyes, "what the HELL kind of title is that? It doesn't tell me what you did or what you found. It doesn't even tell me what you studied, and it sure doesn't make me want to read your paper."

Eight pairs of doctoral student eyes got wide, and we exchanged shocked glances. We didn't notice that the faculty were unfazed. Charlie acknowledged the comment: "Thanks, Don. That's a great point, and I'll work on a more informative and catchy title." Charlie scribbled something in his notebook, and I figured it included some words not suitable for print here.

On the next slide, Charlie introduced the main construct under investigation, and another senior faculty hand shot up. "Of all the things in the world, why would you want to study THAT? Who cares?" This sharp criticism went on for an hour and a half, after which the students convened in our cube farm. "Charlie sure got beat up in there. He must be humiliated." Another said, "Yeah, I thought he was a really good researcher." We all wondered about Charlie's reaction and sent the boldest among us to go find out. He came racing down the hall five minutes later. "You're not going to believe this, but Charlie said it went great. He said he got some great ideas, and he was so lucky to have that group loan him their brainpower for a while. He must be delusional." Confused, we sent our bold colleague off to talk to a senior faculty member. He came back looking even more confused. "You're really not going to believe this, but Barry said the presentation was great, Charlie's really smart, and the paper is sure to find a home in a top journal."

Everyone in that room (except us students) knew about the shared respect and trust among the faculty. Everyone but us knew that Charlie was respected and that hearing these criticisms now would help him produce a manuscript more likely to survive the scrutiny of journal reviewers. Not understanding that made us misconstrue criticism as *judgmental relationship conflict* instead of the constructive task *conflict* it was.

Motivate Your Team Around a Common Purpose

Teams work best when members keep each other motivated and engaged in the work (Chen & Kanfer, 2006; Marks et al., 2001; Van Iddekinge et al., 2018). Group identification and cohesiveness together encourage teammates to work for each other as well as for themselves (Beal et al., 2003; Chang & Bordia, 2001; Stogdill, 1972). Group identification makes outcomes more valuable to each teammate. It also drives members to work hard and compensate for the underperformance of others (Fishbach et al., 2011).

Crisis Phase Conclusions

When the crisis phase starts, good leaders assess their resources. They plan to compensate for weaknesses when possible. They closely monitor environmental pressure on their team members. They maintain positive communication and motivation, and they actively manage conflicts in taskwork and teamwork, all of which can get lost in a crisis.

The Post-Crisis Phase

Crises reveal a team's strengths and weaknesses, provide members with intense, shared experiences, and can help teams prepare for the next event. Post-crisis is the time to take a breath, reassess, and attend to healing and recovery. It is also a chance to evaluate the team's mental state, consolidate learnings, and prepare for future challenges.

Frame the Experience

Learning from crisis starts by recognizing the learning opportunity as a team. In fact, promoting a learning focus even during the crisis can make teams more adaptable (LePine, 2005). Leaders can guide the learning during the post-crisis period using the framework of flexible (easy things to change) and glacial (must be built over time) resources to highlight performance wins and losses, then lead a review emphasizing strengthening of glacial states.

Debrief the Crisis

Researchers have found that retrospective assessments, or "debriefs," similar to root cause analyses in the healthcare context (Lacerenza et al., 2018), improve many team outcomes (Keiser & Arthur, 2021; Tannenbaum & Cerasoli, 2013). Characteristics of effective debriefs include using an objective recall aid such as video or notes, rather than relying on the memory of participants (Villado & Arthur, 2013), conducting debriefs with co-located rather than geographically distributed or virtual teams (Jarrett et al., 2016), and focusing thematically on performance and teamwork aspects of the crisis rather than reviewing events in a chronological order (Lacerenza et al., 2018). Self-led and expert-led debriefs perform equally well, and highly structured debriefs provide no advantage in healthcare settings (Keiser & Arthur, 2021).

Amass External Resources

Debriefs should focus on easily changeable resources and might include adjusting or creating new team roles with an eye toward ongoing (non-crisis) team performance. Since each crisis requires unique structural changes, leaders should carefully consider whether permanently increasing the number or effort of team members, infrastructure, or financial resources is needed when crises are rare. The broader organizational strategy literature suggests that carrying a modest amount of "slack" resources, in the form of financial reserves, can be beneficial (Zona, 2012) while operating significantly below capacity in other ways provides less benefit (Tan & Peng, 2003).

Mitigate the Emotional Impact of the Crisis

The post-crisis phase presents an opportunity for recovery. Alongside the relief of having withstood the crisis, your team may feel emotionally drained, burned out, and stressed. Simply acknowledging the stresses and needs of your team relieves some stress and lets them know they are not alone. Group debrief sessions reinforce the common experience and give your team a chance to process their feelings. You might offer grief counseling or communicate information about employee assistance programs.

Post-Crisis Phase Conclusions

In the post-crisis phase, use a structured process to learn how to manage the next crisis and decide on the resources that you will need to be best prepared in the future. Take time to assess the emotional status of your team members. Offer team members empathy, the opportunity to talk about how they feel, and resources to promote recovery. On an optimistic note, team belongingness and community cohesion can provide emotional resilience, less depression and mood disturbance, and lower levels of "compassion fatigue" and burnout (Henderson et al., 1998; Wu et al., 2016). Successfully working together through a crisis may build a stronger team.

Citations

Acton, B. P., Braun, M. T., & Foti, R. J. (2020). Built for Unity: Assessing the Impact of Team Composition on Team Cohesion Trajectories. *Journal of Business and Psychology, 35*(6), 751-766. https://doi.org/10.1007/s10869-019-09654-7

Baard, S. K., Rench, T. A., & Kozlowski, S. W. J. (2014). Performance Adaptation: A Theoretical Integration and Review. *Journal of Management, 40*(1), 48-99. https://doi.org/10.1177/0149206313488210

Bass, B. M. (1999). Two Decades of Research and Development in Transformational Leadership. *European Journal of Work and Organizational Psychology, 8*(1), 9-32. https://doi.org/10.1080/135943299398410

Beal, D. J., Cohen, R. R., Burke, M. J., & McLendon, C. L. (2003). Cohesion and Performance in Groups: A Meta-Analytic Clarification of Construct Relations. *Journal of Applied Psychology, 88*(6), 989-1004. https://doi.org/10.1037/0021-9010.88.6.989

Bienefeld, N., & Grote, G. (2014). Speaking up in Ad hoc Multiteam Systems: Individual-level Effects of Psychological Safety, Status, and Leadership within and across Teams. *European Journal of Work and Organizational Psychology, 23*(6), 930-945. https://doi.org/10.1080/1359432X.2013.808398

Brandon, D. P., & Hollingshead, A. B. (2004). Transactive Memory Systems in Organizations: Matching Tasks, Expertise, and People. *Organization Science, 15*(6), 633-644. https://doi.org/10.1287/orsc.1040.0069

Cannon-Bowers, J. A., Salas, E., and Converse, S. (1993). Shared Mental Models in Expert Team Decision Making. In N. J. Castellan (Ed.), *Individual and Group Decision Making: Current Issues*. Psychology Press.

Carroll, G. R., & Hannan, M. T. (1989). Density Delay in the Evolution of Organizational Populations: A Model and Five Empirical Tests. *Administrative Science Quarterly, 34*(3), 411-430. https://doi.org/10.2307/2393151

Chang, A., & Bordia, P. (2001). A Multidimensional Approach to the Group Cohesion-Group Performance Relationship. *Small Group Research, 32*(4), 379-405. https://doi.org/10.1177/104649640103200401

Chen, G., & Kanfer, R. (2006). Toward a Systems Theory of Motivated Behavior in Work Teams. *Research in Organizational Behavior, 27*, 223-267. https://doi.org/https://doi.org/10.1016/S0191-3085(06)27006-0

Clarke, S. (2015, July 9). Eight Examples of Great Teamwork at the Tour de France. *Cycling Weekly*. https://www.cyclingweekly.com/news/racing/tour-de-france/eight-examples-of-great-teamwork-at-the-tour-de-france-181392

Courtright, S. H., McCormick, B. W., Mistry, S., & Wang, J. (2017). Quality Charters or Quality Members? A Control Theory Perspective on Team Charters and Team Performance. *J Appl Psychol, 102*(10), 1462-1470. https://doi.org/10.1037/apl0000229

Crawford, E. R., & LePine, J. A. (2013). A Configural Theory of Team Processes: Accounting for the Structure of Taskwork and Teamwork. *Academy of Management Review, 38*(1), 32-48. https://doi.org/10.5465/amr.2011.0206

de Wit, F. R. C., Greer, L. L., & Jehn, K. A. (2012). The Paradox of Intragroup Conflict: A Meta-Analysis. *Journal of Applied Psychology, 97*, 360-390. https://doi.org/10.1037/a0024844

DeChurch, L. A., & Mesmer-Magnus, J. R. (2010). Measuring Shared Team Mental Models: A Meta-Analysis. *Group Dynamics: Theory, Research, and Practice, 14*, 1-14. https://doi.org/10.1037/a0017455

Drach-Zahavy, A., & Freund, A. (2007). Team Effectiveness Under Stress: A Structural Contingency Approach. *Journal of Organizational Behavior, 28*(4), 423-450. https://doi.org/https://doi.org/10.1002/job.430

Driskell, J. E., Salas, E., & Driskell, T. (2018). Foundations of Teamwork and Collaboration. *American Psychologist, 73*(4), 334-348. https://doi.org/https://doi.org/10.1037/amp0000241

Driskell, T., Salas, E., & Driskell, J. E. (2018). Teams in Extreme Environments: Alterations in Team Development and Teamwork. *Human Resource Management Review, 28*(4), 434-449. https://doi.org/https://doi.org/10.1016/j.hrmr.2017.01.002

Edmondson, A. (1999). Psychological Safety and Learning Behavior in Work Teams. *Administrative Science Quarterly, 44*(2), 350-383. https://doi.org/10.2307/2666999

Edmondson, A. C., & Lei, Z. (2014). Psychological Safety: The History, Renaissance, and Future of an Interpersonal Construct. *Annual Review of Organizational Psychology and Organizational Behavior, 1*(1), 23-43. https://doi.org/10.1146/annurev-orgpsych-031413-091305

Ellis, A. P. J., Hollenbeck, J. R., Ilgen, D. R., Porter, C. O. L. H., West, B. J., & Moon, H. (2003). Team Learning: Collectively Connecting the Dots. *Journal of Applied Psychology, 88*, 821-835. https://doi.org/10.1037/0021-9010.88.5.821

Entin, E. E., & Serfaty, D. (1999). Adaptive Team Coordination. *Human Factors, 41*(2), 312-325. https://doi.org/10.1518/001872099779591196

Fishbach, A., Henderson, M. D., & Koo, M. (2011). Pursuing Goals with Others: Group Identification and Motivation Resulting from Things Done Versus Things Left Undone. *J Exp Psychol Gen, 140*(3), 520-534. https://doi.org/10.1037/a0023907

Fisher, D. M. (2014). Distinguishing between Taskwork and Teamwork Planning in Teams: Relations with Coordination and Interpersonal Processes. *J Appl Psychol, 99*(3), 423-436. https://doi.org/10.1037/a0034625

Fisher, R. J., & Wakefield, K. (1998). Factors Leading to Group Identification: A Field Study of Winners and Losers. *Psychology & Marketing, 15*(1), 23-40. https://doi.org/https://doi.org/10.1002/(SICI)1520-6793(199801)15:1<23::AID-MAR3>3.0.CO;2-P

Frazier, M. L., Fainshmidt, S., Klinger, R. L., Pezeshkan, A., & Vracheva, V. (2017). Psychological Safety: A Meta-Analytic Review and Extension. *Personnel Psychology, 70*(1), 113-165. https://doi.org/https://doi.org/10.1111/peps.12183

Gross, N., & Martin, W. E. (1952). On Group Cohesiveness. *American Journal of Sociology, 57*(6), 546-564. https://doi.org/10.1086/221041

Han, G., & Harms, P. D. (2010). Team Identification, Trust and Conflict: A Mediation Model. *International Journal of Conflict Management, 21*, 20-43. https://doi.org/10.1108/10444061011016614

Hausknecht, J. P., Trevor, C. O., & Howard, M. J. (2009). Unit-Level Voluntary Turnover Rates and Customer Service Quality: Implications of Group Cohesiveness, Newcomer Concentration, and Size. *J Appl Psychol, 94*(4), 1068-1075. https://doi.org/10.1037/a0015898

Henderson, J., Bourgeois, A. E., Leunes, A., & Meyers, M. C. (1998). Group Cohesiveness, Mood Disturbance, and Stress in Female Basketball Players. *Small Group Research, 29*(2), 212-225. https://doi.org/10.1177/1046496498292004

Henry, K. B., Arrow, H., & Carini, B. (1999). A Tripartite Model of Group Identification: Theory and Measurement. *Small Group Research, 30*(5), 558-581. https://doi.org/10.1177/104649649903000504

Hogg, M. A., Sherman, D. K., Dierselhuis, J., Maitner, A. T., & Moffitt, G. (2007). Uncertainty, Entitativity, and Group Identification. *Journal of Experimental Social Psychology, 43*(1), 135-142. https://doi.org/https://doi.org/10.1016/j.jesp.2005.12.008

Homan, A. C., van Knippenberg, D., Van Kleef, G. A., & De Dreu, C. K. W. (2007). Interacting Dimensions of Diversity: Cross-Categorization and the Functioning of Diverse Work Groups. *Group Dynamics: Theory, Research, and Practice, 11*(2), 79-94. https://doi.org/https://doi.org/10.1037/1089-2699.11.2.79

Hughes, A. M., Gregory, M. E., Joseph, D. L., Sonesh, S. C., Marlow, S. L., Lacerenza, C. N., Benishek, L. E., King, H. B., & Salas, E. (2016). Saving Lives: A Meta-Analysis of Team Training in Healthcare. *Journal of Applied Psychology, 101*(9), 1266-1304. https://doi.org/10.1037/apl0000120

Ilgen, D. R., Hollenbeck, J. R., Johnson, M., & Jundt, D. (2005). Teams in Organizations: From Input-Process-Output Models to IMOI Models. *Annu Rev Psychol, 56*, 517-543. https://doi.org/10.1146/annurev.psych.56.091103.070250

Jarrett, S. M., Glaze, R. M., Schurig, I., Muñoz, G. J., Naber, A. M., McDonald, J. N., Bennett, W., & Arthur, W. (2016). The Comparative Effectiveness of Distributed and Colocated Team After-Action Reviews. *Human Performance, 29*(5), 408-427. https://doi.org/10.1080/08959285.2016.1208662

Jarvenpaa, S. L., Knoll, K., & Leidner, D. E. (1998). Is Anybody Out There? Antecedents of Trust in Global Virtual Teams. *Journal of Management Information Systems, 14*(4), 29-64. https://doi.org/10.1080/07421222.1998.11518185

Jehn, K. A., & Mannix, E. A. (2001). The Dynamic Nature of Conflict: A Longitudinal Study of Intragroup Conflict and Group Performance. *Academy of Management Journal, 44*(2), 238-251. https://doi.org/10.5465/3069453

Jung, D. I., & Sosik, J. J. (2002). Transformational Leadership in Work Groups: The Role of Empowerment, Cohesiveness, and Collective-Efficacy on Perceived Group Performance. *Small Group Research, 33*(3), 313-336. https://doi.org/10.1177/10496402033003002

Keiser, N. L., & Arthur, W. (2021). A Meta-Analysis of the Effectiveness of the After-Action Review (or Debrief) and Factors that Influence its Effectiveness. *J Appl Psychol, 106*(7), 1007-1032. https://doi.org/10.1037/apl0000821

Kent, D., & Granqvist, N. (2020). From Clear Skies to EF5s: How Storm Chasing Teams Stay Engaged with Temporally Uncertain Work. *Academy of Management Proceedings, 2020*, 16715. https://doi.org/10.5465/AMBPP.2020.16715abstract

Korsgaard, M. A., Brower, H. H., & Lester, S. W. (2015). It Isn't Always Mutual: A Critical Review of Dyadic Trust. *Journal of Management, 41*(1), 47-70. https://doi.org/10.1177/0149206314547521

Lacerenza, C. N., Marlow, S. L., Tannenbaum, S. I., & Salas, E. (2018). Team Development Interventions: Evidence-Based Approaches for Improving Teamwork. *American Psychologist, 73*, 517-531. https://doi.org/10.1037/amp0000295

LePine, J. A. (2003). Team Adaptation and Postchange Performance: Effects of Team Composition in Terms of Members' Cognitive Ability and Personality. *J Appl Psychol, 88*(1), 27-39. https://doi.org/10.1037/0021-9010.88.1.27

LePine, J. A. (2005). Adaptation of Teams in Response to Unforeseen Change: Effects of Goal Difficulty and Team Composition in Terms of Cognitive Ability and Goal Orientation. *J Appl Psychol, 90*(6), 1153-1167. https://doi.org/10.1037/0021-9010.90.6.1153

Maltarich, M. A., Kukenberger, M., Reilly, G., & Mathieu, J. (2018). Conflict in Teams: Modeling Early and Late Conflict States and the Interactive Effects of Conflict Processes. *Group & Organization Management, 43*(1), 6-37. https://doi.org/10.1177/1059601116681127

Marks, M. A., Mathieu, J. E., & Zaccaro, S. J. (2001). A Temporally Based Framework and Taxonomy of Team Processes. *The Academy of Management Review, 26*(3), 356-376. https://doi.org/10.2307/259182

Marlow, S. L., Lacerenza, C. N., Paoletti, J., Burke, C. S., & Salas, E. (2018). Does Team Communication Represent a One-Size-Fits-All Approach?: A Meta-Analysis of Team Communication and Performance. *Organizational Behavior and Human Decision Processes, 144*, 145-170. https://doi.org/https://doi.org/10.1016/j.obhdp.2017.08.001

Martin, J. C., Davidson, C. J., & Pardyjak, E. R. (2007). Understanding Sprint-Cycling Performance: The Integration of Muscle Power, Resistance, and Modeling. *Int J Sports Physiol Perform, 2*(1), 5-21. https://doi.org/10.1123/ijspp.2.1.5

Mathieu, J. E., Heffner, T. S., Goodwin, G. F., Salas, E., & Cannon-Bowers, J. A. (2000). The Influence of Shared Mental Models on Team Process and Performance. *Journal of Applied Psychology, 85*, 273-283. https://doi.org/10.1037/0021-9010.85.2.273

Mathieu, J. E., Hollenbeck, J. R., van Knippenberg, D., & Ilgen, D. R. (2017). A Century of Work Teams in the Journal of Applied Psychology. *Journal of Applied Psychology, 102*, 452-467. https://doi.org/10.1037/apl0000128

Mathieu, J. E., Kukenberger, M. R., D'Innocenzo, L., & Reilly, G. (2015). Modeling Reciprocal Team Cohesion-Performance Relationships, as Impacted by Shared Leadership and Members' Competence. *J Appl Psychol, 100*(3), 713-734. https://doi.org/10.1037/a0038898

Mathieu, J. E., & Rapp, T. L. (2009). Laying the Foundation for Successful Team Performance Trajectories: The Roles of Team Charters and Performance Strategies. *J Appl Psychol, 94*(1), 90-103. https://doi.org/10.1037/a0013257

Mathieu, J. E., Tannenbaum, S. I., Kukenberger, M. R., Donsbach, J. S., & Alliger, G. M. (2015). Team Role Experience and Orientation: A Measure and Tests of Construct Validity. *Group & Organization Management, 40*(1), 6-34. https://doi.org/10.1177/1059601114562000

Mayer, R. C., Davis, J. H., & Schoorman, F. D. (1995). An Integrative Model of Organizational Trust. *The Academy of Management Review, 20*(3), 709-734. https://doi.org/10.2307/258792

Maynard, M. T., Kennedy, D. M., & Sommer, S. A. (2015). Team Adaptation: A Fifteen-Year Synthesis (1998–2013) and Framework for how this Literature Needs to "Adapt" Going Forward. *European Journal of Work and Organizational Psychology, 24*(5), 652-677. https://doi.org/10.1080/1359432X.2014.1001376

McAllister, D. J., Lewicki, R. J., & Chaturvedi, S. (2006). Trust in Developing Relationships: From Theory to Measurement. *Academy of Management Proceedings, 2006*(1), G1-G6. https://doi.org/10.5465/ambpp.2006.22897235

McComb, S., & Simpson, V. (2014). The Concept of Shared Mental Models in Healthcare Collaboration. *Journal of Advanced Nursing, 70*(7), 1479-1488. https://doi.org/https://doi.org/10.1111/jan.12307

Meister, A., Thatcher, S. M. B., Park, J., & Maltarich, M. (2020). Toward A Temporal Theory of Faultlines and Subgroup Entrenchment. *Journal of Management Studies, 57*(8), 1473-1501. https://doi.org/https://doi.org/10.1111/joms.12538

Mesmer-Magnus, J. R., & DeChurch, L. A. (2009). Information Sharing and Team Performance: A Meta-Analysis. *Journal of Applied Psychology, 94*, 535-546. https://doi.org/10.1037/a0013773

Miller, A. J., Slater, M. J., & Turner, M. J. (2020). Coach Identity Leadership Behaviours Are Positively Associated with Athlete Resource Appraisals: The Mediating Roles of Relational and Group Identification. *Psychology of Sport and Exercise, 51*, 101755. https://doi.org/https://doi.org/10.1016/j.psychsport.2020.101755

Mishra, A. K. (1996). Organizational Responses to Crisis: The Centrality of Trust. In R. M. a. T. Kramer, T.R. (Ed.), *Trust in Organizations: Frontiers of Theory and Research* (pp. 261-287). Sage.

Newman, A., Donohue, R., & Eva, N. (2017). Psychological Safety: A Systematic Review of the Literature. *Human Resource Management Review, 27*(3), 521-535. https://doi.org/https://doi.org/10.1016/j.hrmr.2017.01.001

O'Neill, O. A. (2009). Workplace Expression of Emotions and Escalation of Commitment. *Journal of Applied Social Psychology, 39*(10), 2396-2424. https://doi.org/https://doi.org/10.1111/j.1559-1816.2009.00531.x

Olie, R., Klijn, E., & Leenders, H. (2020). United or Divided? Antecedents of Board Cohesiveness in International Joint Ventures. *Academy of Management Proceedings, 2020*(1), 21123. https://doi.org/10.5465/ambpp.2020.29

Peltokorpi, V. (2008). Transactive Memory Systems. *Review of General Psychology, 12*(4), 378-394. https://doi.org/10.1037/1089-2680.12.4.378

Ren, Y., & Argote, L. (2011). Transactive Memory Systems 1985–2010: An Integrative Framework of Key Dimensions, Antecedents, and Consequences. *Academy of Management Annals, 5*(1), 189-229. https://doi.org/10.5465/19416520.2011.590300

Roethlisberger, F. J., & Dickson, W. J. (1939). *Management and the Worker*. Harvard Univ. Press.

Rouse, W. B., & Morris, N. M. (1986). On Looking into the Black Box: Prospects and Limits in the Search for Mental Models. *Psychological Bulletin, 100*, 349-363. https://doi.org/10.1037/0033-2909.100.3.349

Salas, E., Cooke, N. J., & Rosen, M. A. (2008). On Teams, Teamwork, and Team Performance: Discoveries and Developments. *Human Factors, 50*(3), 540-547. https://doi.org/10.1518/001872008x288457

Salas, E., Wilson, K. A., Burke, C. S., & Wightman, D. C. (2006). Does Crew Resource Management Training Work? An update, an extension, and some critical needs. *Hum Factors, 48*(2), 392-412. https://doi.org/10.1518/001872006777724444

Seong, J. Y., Kristof-Brown, A. L., Park, W.-W., Hong, D.-S., & Shin, Y. (2015). Person-Group Fit: Diversity Antecedents, Proximal Outcomes, and Performance at the Group Level. *Journal of Management, 41*(4), 1184-1213. https://doi.org/10.1177/0149206312453738

Sexton, K., Johnson, A., Gotsch, A., Hussein, A. A., Cavuoto, L., & Guru, K. A. (2018). Anticipation, Teamwork and Cognitive Load: Chasing Efficiency during Robot-Assisted Surgery. B*MJ Quality & Safety, 27*(2), 148. https://doi.org/10.1136/bmjqs-2017-006701

Simsek, Z., Fox, B. C., & Heavey, C. (2015). "What's Past Is Prologue": A Framework, Review, and Future Directions for Organizational Research on Imprinting. *Journal of Management, 41*(1), 288-317. https://doi.org/10.1177/0149206314553276

Stachowski, A. A., Kaplan, S. A., & Waller, M. J. (2009). The Benefits of Flexible Team Interaction during Crises. *J Appl Psychol, 94*(6), 1536-1543. https://doi.org/10.1037/a0016903

Steiner, I. D. (1972). *Group Process and Productivity*. Academic Press New York.

Stewart, G. L., Courtright, S. H., & Barrick, M. R. (2012). Peer-Based Control in Self-Managing Teams: Linking Rational and Normative Influence with Individual and Group Performance. *J Appl Psychol, 97*(2), 435-447. https://doi.org/10.1037/a0025303

Stogdill, R. M. (1972). Group Productivity, Drive, and Cohesiveness. *Organizational Behavior and Human Performance, 8*(1), 26-43. https://doi.org/https://doi.org/10.1016/0030-5073(72)90035-9

Sverdrup, T. E., Schei, V., & Tjølsen, Ø. A. (2017). Expecting the Unexpected: Using Team Charters to Handle Disruptions and Facilitate Team Performance. *Group Dynamics: Theory, Research, and Practice, 21*, 53-59. https://doi.org/10.1037/gdn0000059

Tan, J., & Peng, M. W. (2003). Organizational Slack and Firm Performance during Economic Transitions: Two Studies from an Emerging Economy. *Strategic Management Journal, 24*(13), 1249-1263. https://doi.org/https://doi.org/10.1002/smj.351

Tziner, A., & Eden, D. (1985). Effects of Crew Composition on Crew Performance: Does the Whole Equal the Sum of its Parts? *Journal of Applied Psychology, 70*, 85-93. https://doi.org/10.1037/0021-9010.70.1.85

Van Iddekinge, C. H., Aguinis, H., Mackey, J. D., & DeOrtentiis, P. S. (2018). A Meta-Analysis of the Interactive, Additive, and Relative Effects of Cognitive Ability and Motivation on Performance. *Journal of Management, 44*(1), 249-279. https://doi.org/10.1177/0149206317702220

van Knippenberg, D., Haslam, S. A., & Platow, M. J. (2007). Unity through Diversity: Value-in-Diversity Beliefs, Work Group Diversity, and Group Identification. *Group Dynamics: Theory, Research, and Practice, 11*, 207-222. https://doi.org/10.1037/1089-2699.11.3.207

Villado, A. J., & Arthur, W., Jr. (2013). The Comparative Effect of Subjective and Objective After-action Reviews on Team Performance on a Complex Task. *Journal of Applied Psychology, 98*(3), 514–528. https://doi.org/10.1037/a0031510

Wolfson, M. A., & Mathieu, J. E. (2018). Sprinting to the Finish: Toward a Theory of Human Capital Resource Complementarity. *J Appl Psychol, 103*(11), 1165-1180. https://doi.org/10.1037/apl0000323

Wolfson, M. A., & Mathieu, J. E. (2021). Deploying Human Capital Resources: Accentuating Effects of Situational Alignment and Social Capital Resources. *Academy of Management Journal, 64*(2), 435-457.

Wu, S., Singh-Carlson, S., Odell, A., Reynolds, G., & Su, Y. (2016). Compassion Fatigue, Burnout, and Compassion Satisfaction Among Oncology Nurses in the United States and Canada. *Oncol Nurs Forum, 43*(4), E161-169. https://doi.org/10.1188/16.Onf.E161-e169

Yun, S., Faraj, S., & Sims, H. P., Jr. (2005). Contingent Leadership and Effectiveness of Trauma Resuscitation Teams. *J Appl Psychol, 90*(6), 1288-1296. https://doi.org/10.1037/0021-9010.90.6.1288

Zona, F. (2012). Corporate Investing as a Response to Economic Downturn: Prospect Theory, the Behavioural Agency Model and the Role of Financial Slack. *British Journal of Management, 23*(S1), S42-S57. https://doi.org/https://doi.org/10.1111/j.1467-8551.2012.00818.x

CHAPTER 2

Practical Applications of the Conceptual Framework:
How to Lead Your Team Through a Crisis

Mark A. Maltarich, PhD

Darla Moore School of Business, University of South Carolina

Kathlyn E. Fletcher, MD, MA

Medical College of Wisconsin

Nothing is as practical as a good theory.

—Kurt Lewin, 1945, p. 129

In this chapter, the authors elaborate on the conceptual framework presented in Chapter 1. The authors illustrate the framework's ideas through examples and offer practical suggestions for leaders to use during the pre-crisis, crisis, and post-crisis phases.

Introduction

The framework offered in Chapter 1 breaks a crisis into three periods (pre-crisis, crisis, and post-crisis), each with different key actions. The framework makes explicit that the pre-crisis phase is the time to focus on building your team. Some parts of building your team are flexible and could be adapted in the crisis phase, including who is on your team, what their roles are, and how you are organized. The pre-crisis phase is also the time to develop "glacial" or slow-to-build team resources such as trust, shared mental models of the work, deep organizational knowledge, cohesiveness, group identification, and psychological safety. In the crisis phase, you will assess those team resources and make plans to overcome deficits. You will concentrate on communication, managing conflict within the team, and motivating them. In the post-crisis phase, you will focus on recovering and rebuilding through debriefing, framing the experience, asking for needed resources to perform better in the next crisis, helping your team recover emotionally from the crisis, and working together to strengthen your team.

Practical Wisdom and Advice in the Pre-Crisis Phase

Well begun is half done.
—Anonymous

In the pre-crisis phase, when the work is relatively predictable and the team is functioning well, you may assume that you don't need to change anything. You might not notice problems with structure, process, and relationships. Remember that every stable period could be the calm before the next storm, so use the pre-crisis time wisely to develop favorable task work, teamwork, and glacial team resources.

Recognize phases and transitions and communicate them to the team
The first step is to recognize which crisis phase you are in and communicate it to the team to ensure you all get on the same page (recall the storm chasers from Chapter 1). As the COVID-19 pandemic spread rapidly around the globe, hospitals effectively signaled the transition from the pre-crisis to the crisis phase through the creation of crisis-steering committees and policy changes to prevent transmission within the hospital. These changes signaled to hospital staff that a crisis had begun (Kent & Granqvist, 2020). However, pinpointing the transition to the post-crisis phase of COVID-19 has been more difficult. In fact, we observed several "mini-cycles" in the COVID-19 crisis as different virus variants surged. The federal government officially declared the pandemic over in May 2023, a signal that we had moved to the post-crisis phase. Since GME leaders will interact differently with their teams depending on the crisis phase, build good systems for gathering information about potential crises and establishing a communication strategy for transitions.

Build a common understanding of the environment, team, and mission (shared mental model) through articulating shared values in your everyday work
The relative predictability of the pre-crisis phase allows leaders the luxury to reflect on their

core values and solidify the principles that will guide their actions during a crisis. Communicating these values sets the culture and moral compass for the team, makes for more effective ethical leadership, and discourages dysfunctional team behaviors (Mayer et al., 2012). *Atomic Habits*, by James Clear, offers a strategy for starting with small actions toward living out your values as an individual or a team (Clear, 2018).

Leaders can prepare for any crisis by building shared mental models about core values and how they influence goals, strategies, and key success factors through routine communication (Table 1). For example, curiosity is a core value in our (KF's) leadership group. We try to live by Ted Lasso's maxim of "be curious, not judgmental" in our approach to resident concerns. In 2021–2022, the residents began a discussion with us about being allowed to "moonlight" or work outside of their residency responsibilities for extra money. The leadership team opposed moonlighting because we had made extensive changes to reduce resident hours at work for well-being (and accreditation) purposes. In July 2022, after months of discussion, the residents sent me a formal proposal making the argument that financial well-being impacted overall well-being. We approached their request with curiosity. In a regular leadership meeting, we debated the pros and cons of allowing moonlighting and gave the residents a counterproposal that limited how much and when moonlighting could occur. Residents expressed gratitude at being heard. The compromise plan was implemented, and third-year residents in good standing were allowed to moonlight. Using core values—in this case, curiosity instead of judgment—will make the next challenge in routine decision-making easier for the leadership group.

Table 1. Routine strategies for building shared mental models through core values
- Agree on core values within the leadership group
- Name the core values when they arise in routine decision-making
- Include time on meeting agendas for discussion of core values, strategies to demonstrate them, and check-ins to hold the team accountable
- Create official onboarding and/or recurrent required training that highlights core values

Allow the past to help inform the future during regular meetings and informal conversations

A program's cultural information is strongly communicated in stories, myths, and legends about past crises and organizational actors (Duncan, 1989; Martin, 2016). Sharing your program's history and creating opportunities for others to share and process stories serve to create deep organizational knowledge. In regularly scheduled meetings, team members may propose ideas that have been tried in the past without success. Linking past failure with a story can connect newer team members with the history and can also generate discussion to make the idea successful. For example, every year, we have discussions about how to manage absences in September and October when senior residents are interviewing for fellowships. Someone always mentions that residents usually attend a moderate number of interviews (and therefore maybe we don't need to have a specific policy). However, one year we had a resident miss 22 days in a single month for interviews. We laugh, roll our eyes, and remember why we have rules about such processes.

Use (and intentionally plan) interactions as an opportunity to develop relationships

The pre-crisis phase is an opportunity to develop trust related to teamwork and interpersonal relationships. Exposure to others' tasks and roles gradually builds an understanding of teammates' individual work and how everyone fits together. Indeed, the small talk at the beginning of a meeting may serve such a purpose. Sometimes, small talk is work related, sometimes personal. Such informal connection helps us understand each other's lives. Many of these conversations arise organically, but the leader should notice days when the group needs an intentional effort to promote interactions. I (KF) once began a weekly meeting with the following icebreaker: "What is the thing that you are most worried about right this minute?" Selfishly, I knew that I needed to say my worry out loud to be able to concentrate on the meeting. I was relieved that others shared their concerns too, and the exercise helped us release the worries and support each other. Gatherings aimed at getting to know each other (and each other's families) are good for building relationships and a sense of belonging, especially when new team members are added to the group.

Deliberately build psychological safety and group identification

Psychological safety stems from supportive and inclusive leadership at all levels and recognized similarities among teammates (Newman et al., 2017). A study in the healthcare setting (Nembhard & Edmondson, 2006) found that the social status healthcare workers derive from their profession was positively associated with psychological safety, suggesting that leaders might help junior members of the leadership team speak up by highlighting and reinforcing their status, professionalism, and accomplishments.

Leaders should promote group identification. Group efficacy—collective belief in the team's capability to succeed—is an antecedent of group identification (van Zomeren et al., 2010), suggesting that celebrating wins is an effective way to build positive team states. An experienced and knowledgeable leader expressing confidence in the team can go a long way toward building their own self-confidence (Bandura, 1977). Regular meetings provide an opportunity to highlight small wins. For example, we routinely have updates on intern recruitment during our weekly meetings in October through January. We intentionally discuss things that are going well and praise the APDs and program staff in charge of recruitment. During resident retreats, our APD for Wellness hands out sticky notes for the residents to write what they are grateful

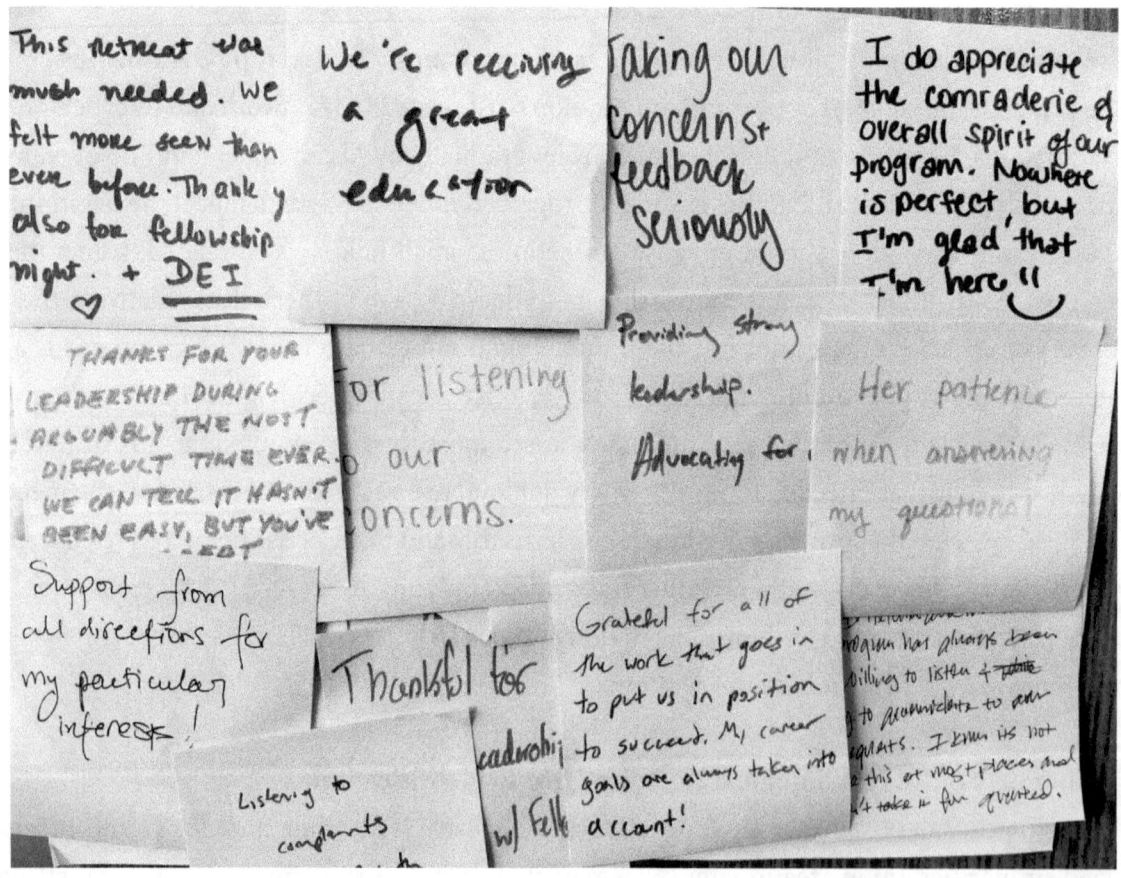

for about our program staff, chief residents, and program as a whole. She displays the sticky notes afterwards as a daily reminder of how we each contribute to the success of our program.

Assess your team

Despite some skepticism about their application to healthcare settings (Floren et al., 2018), it is possible to measure concepts like shared mental models (DeChurch & Mesmer-Magnus, 2010), cultural values and norms (Hofstede et al., 1990; Ostroff et al., 2005) and tracking team convergence (Fulmer & Ostroff, 2016; Lang et al., 2018). If you are interested in measuring key team states and tracking them (and the team's agreement on them) over time, these tools (Table 2) are readily available and low cost in terms of both time and money. Many of the cited publications include full lists of scale items and information about typical distributions of scores, though usually in a limited population or context.

<<*Figure. Sticky notes of gratitude written by residents to their program leadership.*

Table 2. Important constructs from the conceptual framework and tools for measuring them

	Construct	Measure	Source(s)
Resources	Team Roles	TREO	Mathieu et al., 2015
	Structure	Shared leadership	Zhu et al., 2018
		Decentralization	Hollenbeck et al., 2011
	Personnel	Quantity and quality	Nyberg et al., 2014
	Trust	Propensity to trust	Frazier et al., 2013
		Intrateam trust	de Jong & Elfring, 2010; Feitosa et al., 2020
	Deep Organizational Knowledge	TMS	Lewis, 2003
	Shared Mental Models	Cue-strategy association measure	Smith-Jentsch et al., 2005
		QAP Matrix Correlation	Mathieu et al., 2000
	Cohesiveness	Group Environment Questionnaire	Chang & Bordia, 2000; Seashore, 1954
	Group Identification	Group identification	Henry et al., 1999
		In-group identification	Leach et al., 2008
	Psychological Safety	Team psychological safety	Edmondson, 1999

Processes	Communication	Anticipation ratio	Sexton et al., 2018 Stachowski et al., 2009
		Communication and Teamwork Skills (CATS) assessment	Frankel et al., 2007
	Coordination	Judged by observation	Shah & Breazeal, 2010
	Conflict	Task, relationship, and process conflict scale	Jehn & Mannix, 2001
	Conflict Management	Conflict styles scales	Rahim, 1983
		Conflict responses scales	De Dreu et al., 2001
		Conflict management approaches	Chen & Tjosvold, 2005

Note: We selected these references based on the degree to which the scale is relied upon in high-quality teams research, the free availability of scale items, and the ease of implementation. Many other scales are available.

Summary for the Pre-Crisis Phase

In the pre-crisis phase, your focus should be on developing the glacial resources of your program. Regular meetings offer opportunities to define and incorporate program values. You can also design activities and discussions that promote group cohesion, shared mental models, and deep organizational knowledge. If you feel uncertain about your team's status in these glacial resources, consider measuring them so that you can focus your attention on those resources that most need it.

Practical Wisdom and Advice in the Crisis Phase

God, grant me the serenity to accept the things I cannot change, the courage to change the things I can, and the wisdom to know the difference . . .
—Reinhold Niebuhr (in Sifton, 2003)

Assess your team (again)

Crises come suddenly, and there's no time to build trust. It's too late to develop cohesiveness. You can't suddenly make people willing to speak up if they have been routinely ignored or discounted. However, there are work-arounds for some of these problems, and some flexible resources can be changed more readily. Therefore, the first job of the leader is to assess the current state of the team and compare that assessment to the needs of the situation. The measurement strategies in Table 2 can help.

Employ work-arounds for glacial resource weaknesses

Though glacial resources cannot be changed in the short term, recognizing weak points for taskwork or teamwork can suggest specific actions. For example, the termination (firing) of a resident is a crisis heavy in decision-making. Leadership teams that lack psychological safety, have poor conflict norms, or are overly cohesive will struggle to generate alternative courses of action and evaluate them effectively. In the midst of such a crisis, you cannot change these attributes, but as a leader, you are not powerless.

One approach is to use the flexible resources of team process and role structure to the team's advantage. A brainstorming approach, for instance, can help generate alternative ideas in groups that might be expected to struggle. First, ask team members to write their ideas on paper. Next, collect them and write each idea on a board until everyone's full list is represented. Finally, have the group talk through the ideas together (Rossiter & Lilien, 1994).

Another work-around is to explicitly assign a teammate to the role of "devil's advocate" and publicly ask them to be as critical as possible about whatever idea is on the table (Schweiger et al., 1989; Schwenk, 1990). The explicit assignment of such a role ensures that ideas will get a critical evaluation but takes social pressure off the person assigned to be the devil's advocate. The devil's advocate can speak freely, without concern for retribution or hard feelings.

Use purpose as a motivator

Because of the enormous, potential emotional impact of working during a program crisis, leaders must pay attention to teams that might lack social support or mutual motivation. Crises in the medical context have the unique advantage of highlighting the vocational calling and purpose of teams, and leaders can leverage this to keep workers energized and psychologically healthy (Kahn, 1990). The purpose of taking care of patients and residents during such a crisis may be enough motivation, but taking care of each other can also motivate teams. Indeed, in an email to the Medical College of Wisconsin (MCW) community, MCW President Dr. John Raymond specifically noted that he was grateful during the pandemic "to have the privilege to lead our organization at such a critical time." The pandemic brought a unique opportunity for PDs to use purpose as a motivator because healthcare workers were uniquely positioned as critical to public health, and, for a time, the public outpouring of support reflected the deep societal value attached to the work.

In essays written by residents in March of 2020, the theme of work as a calling was already evident (Stevens-Haas, 2021). One resident anonymously wrote, " . . . The real special part is that we can help give time for patients to have what is really important: time to see a grandchild's wedding, time to share holidays; time to have an argument, then reconcile. Doctors can help give patients more time for everything that makes life, life: connection. The science and puzzle-solving and recognition and thanks are all great but the privilege of serving others through medicine is that the work is a shortcut to share some of that connection with every patient . . ." PDs should celebrate and perpetuate the motivation coming directly from the residents.

Tend to the needs of individual team member using empathy and caring
The stress of healthcare work in a crisis carries risks to the physical and mental health of team members. In addition to attending to the interpersonal elements of teamwork, leaders have to take some responsibility for the well-being of individuals. In a national study of internal medicine PDs conducted in August 2020, a prominent theme of early pandemic difficulties focused on the PDs' emotions such as fear, anxiety, stress, and being overwhelmed (Fletcher et al., 2022). They noted feeling responsible for the psychological well-being and the physical well-being of faculty and residents, and indeed many residents were fearful. One wrote anonymously: "I am absolutely certain that I will be infected . . ." (Stevens-Haas, 2021)

These disparate feelings—being motivated by purpose and extremely fearful—existed in leadership teams as well. Being aware of them and tending to both was essential to healthy functioning. In fact, many people felt both emotions simultaneously, or at least in alternating succession. Other crises result in conflicting emotions within and between team members, and strong leaders will recognize that this requires "individualized consideration." Individualized consideration is described (with different labels) in most leadership theories such as leader-member exchange (Buengeler et al., 2021; Henderson et al., 2009; Martin et al., 2016), transformational leadership (Bass, 1999; Rafferty & Griffin, 2006; Wang et al., 2011), and others. Time may be scarce, but acting with genuine concern for each team member can help keep them safe and healthy, motivated and engaged in their work, focused on success and peak performance, and more deeply committed to the team and organization in the future.

Summary for the Crisis Phase

Reassess your team for hard-to build resources like trust. If some are missing, employ work-arounds to ensure optimal decision-making. Try to harness each team member's sense of purpose in the work to motivate them through hard times, especially when the crisis extends for a long period. Finally, employ individualized consideration by meeting people where they are with respect to their fears and needs. Empathy and caring are necessary character traits in crisis.

Practical Wisdom and Advice in the Post-Crisis Phase

Never let a good crisis go to waste.
—Winston Churchill

Nobody hopes for a crisis, but crises offer a stress test for teams and organizations that can expose weak points, suggest improvements, provide shared experiences that can bring teams closer, and identify needed resources. Leveraging a crisis for gain might feel ghoulish, but making the most of what your team learned is good leadership. Here we offer specific advice for managing individual, team-level, and external considerations after the crisis. Doing the right things in the post-crisis phase lays a new foundation for successful operation in the "new normal" period of pre-crisis.

A central tenet of the post-crisis period is that crises have causes that ripple through time, and disruptions usually persist beyond the most acute phase of a crisis until things settle into the new normal of a pre-crisis phase (Pieper et al., 2023; Reilly et al., 2014). Take George Floyd's death and the Black Lives Matter movement (covered in Chapter 6) as an example. The death of George Floyd was the result of centuries of injustice and unequal treatment. The protests shed a brighter light on that injustice, and the medical community continues to wrestle (appropriately) with our own contribution to systemic racism.

Use grace, empathy, and caring to facilitate individual healing

Many team members will have neglected personal needs, obligations, and relationships during the crisis. Depending on the circumstances, some could be affected by post-traumatic stress disorder (PTSD), substance use, or other health issues. We (KF's program) observed a range of reactions in the post-crisis phase of the pandemic within our leadership group, especially around returning to work. Some team members were uncomfortable returning to shared office space and did most administrative work from home. Some wanted to have fully in-person weekly team meetings. By allowing a virtual option, we provided validation for the many paths back to normal. Allowing physical and emotional space for climbing out of the COVID-19 abyss was our team's version of grace.

Recognizing, processing, and attending to your teammates as individuals has the additional benefit of helping to build trust, cohesiveness, and other glacial team resources. Such actions also model the importance of grace, caring, empathy, and compassion as core values to your team and demonstrate that you as the leader believe in these things for them as well as for your residents. Use the opportunity to update your assessments of individuals' strengths and weaknesses, as well as their adaptability and resilience in the face of high pressure. Finally, don't forget the importance of taking care of yourself (see Chapter 10 for ideas).

Focus on team growth opportunities

In addition to helping individual teammates recover, debriefing and assessing the crisis response will help the team understand its strengths and weaknesses. What did the team do well, and why? What could have gone better, and what got in the way? The framework provided in Chapter 1 (Figure 1) can serve as a template for such discussions. For example, you might ask performance questions related to communication, conflict, and motivation. If the group identifies a shortcoming in their response related to communication, the team characteristics offer a menu for diagnosing the underlying issue: Did the communication issues arise because of a structure that was too siloed? Or because of a lack of psychological safety? Or misunderstandings about the roles and responsibilities of others on the team? Making these kinds of very specific attributions should be done as a group, because teammates will have different information, perspectives, and experiences from the crisis. Even though some problems are unlikely to recur, make improvements anyway. This review process provides a road map for team development during the upcoming pre-crisis phase.

Identify resource needs and ask for them

Churchill saw the potential for a crisis to convince external constituents of the need for additional support. What do you need in human capital, financial resources, infrastructure, and technology to be ready for the next crisis? You may need to expand the outward-facing roles of APDs to lobby for resources from your department or hospital system. Hospitals will likely convene their own after-action review committees, so choosing delegates and coordinating strategies will be an important part of the post-crisis work.

Summary for the Post-Crisis Phase

In the post-crisis phase, attend to the individual needs of teammates and the team. Give your teammates time and space to heal in their own ways. Debrief your processes and identify things to work on as a team to be prepared for the next crisis. Celebrate your successes and the shared experiences. Use them to grow closer. Identify resources that will help you in the future and lobby for them.

Table 3: Summary of practical advice		
Phase	Domain	Intervention / Action Items
Pre-Crisis	Assess phases and transitions	• Monitor the environment • Communicate changes • Track flexible and glacial resources
	Build glacial team resources	• Agree on values and priorities • Tell stories about the program's history • Create opportunities to get to know each other • Celebrate small wins
	Measure and track key resources	• Deploy validated surveys • Track levels over time
Crisis	Reassess team	• Measure or judge team resources • Assess the needs of the current crisis
	Adjust to shortcomings	• Put systems in place (work-arounds) to offset weaknesses • Adjust flexible resources
	Attend to teamwork	• Monitor and manage conflict • Communicate to align information, goals, and perceptions • Assign explicit team roles
	Attend to individuals	• Monitor health and well-being • Assign explicit team roles
Post-Crisis	Attend to individuals	• Promote social support • Highlight organizational offerings for mental health • Provide individualized support for recovery
	Attend to the team	• Debrief and highlight shared experiences
	Assess resource needs	• Identify resources needed • Restructure to lobby and acquire new resources

Citations

Bandura, A. (1977). Self-Efficacy: Toward a Unifying Theory of Behavioral Change. *Psychological Review, 84*, 191-215. https://doi.org/10.1037/0033-295X.84.2.191

Bass, B. M. (1999). Two Decades of Research and Development in Transformational Leadership. *European Journal of Work and Organizational Psychology, 8*(1), 9-32. https://doi.org/10.1080/135943299398410

Buengeler, C., Piccolo, R. F., & Locklear, L. R. (2021). LMX Differentiation and Group Outcomes: A Framework and Review Drawing on Group Diversity Insights. *Journal of Management, 47*(1), 260-287. https://doi.org/10.1177/0149206320930813

Chang, A., & Bordia, P. (2001). A Multidimensional Approach to the Group Cohesion-Group Performance Relationship. *Small Group Research, 32*(4), 379-405. https://doi.org/10.1177/104649640103200401

Chen, G., Tjosvold, D. Conflict Management and Team Effectiveness in China: The Mediating Role of Justice. *Asia Pacific Journal of Management 19*, 557-572. https://doi.org/10.1023/A:1020573710461

Clear, J. (2018). *Atomic Habits: An Easy & Proven Way to Build Good Habits & Break Bad Ones*. Avery, an imprint of Penguin Random House. New York, New York.

DeChurch, L. A., & Mesmer-Magnus, J. R. (2010). Measuring Shared Team Mental Models: A Meta-Analysis. *Group Dynamics: Theory, Research, and Practice, 14*, 1-14. https://doi.org/10.1037/a0017455

De Dreu, C., Evers, A., Beersma, B., Kluwer, E. & Nauta, A. (2001). A Theory-Based Measure of Conflict Management in the Workplace. *J Organ Behav, 22*. 645-668. https://doi.org/10.1002/job.107.

De Jong, B.A. & Elfring, T. (2010). How Does Trust Affect the Performance of Ongoing Teams? The Mediating Role of Reflexivity, Monitoring and Effort. *Acad Manage J, 53*, 535-549. https://doi.org/10.5465/amj.2010.51468649

Duncan, W. J. (1989). Organizational Culture: "Getting a Fix" on an Elusive Concept. *Academy of Management Perspectives, 3*(3), 229-236. https://doi.org/10.5465/ame.1989.4274741

Edmondson, A. (1999). Psychological Safety and Learning Behavior in Work Teams. *Administrative Science Quarterly, 44*(2), 350-383. https://doi.org/10.2307/2666999

Feitosa, J., Grossman, R., Kramer, W., & Salas, E. (2020). Measuring Team Trust: A Critical and Meta-Analytical Review. *J Organ Behav, 41*. https://doi.org/10.1002/job.2436

Frankel, A., Gardner, R., Maynard, L., & Kelly, A. (2007). Using the Communication and Teamwork Skills (CATS) Assessment to Measure Health Care Team Performance. *Jt Comm J Qual and Patient Saf, 33*(9), 549-558.

Frazier, M., Johnson, P., & Fainshmidt, S. (2013). Development and Validation of a Propensity to Trust Scale. *Journal of Trust Research, 3*. 76-97. https://doi.org/10.1080/21515581.2013.820026

Floren, L. C., Donesky, D., Whitaker, E., Irby, D. M., Ten Cate, O., & O'Brien, B. C. (2018). Are We on the Same Page? Shared Mental Models to Support Clinical Teamwork Among Health Professions Learners: A Scoping Review. *Acad Med, 93*(3), 498-509. https://doi.org/10.1097/acm.0000000000002019

Fletcher, K. E., Finn, K. M., Kiselewski, M., Simmons, R., Zaas, A., & Zetkulic, M. (September 23, 2022). *The Trauma of the COVID-19 Pandemic: Impact on Residency Program Directors*. Fall Association of Program Directors in Internal Medicine Meeting.

Fulmer, C. A., & Ostroff, C. (2016). Convergence and Emergence in Organizations: An Integrative Framework and Review. *Journal of Organizational Behavior, 37*(S1), S122-S145. https://doi.org/10.1002/job.1987

Henderson, D. J., Liden, R. C., Glibkowski, B. C., & Chaudhry, A. (2009). LMX Differentiation: A Multilevel Review and Examination of its Antecedents and Outcomes. *The Leadership Quarterly, 20*(4), 517-534. https://doi.org/10.1016/j.leaqua.2009.04.003

Henry, K. B., Arrow, H., & Carini, B. (1999). A Tripartite Model of Group Identification:Theory and Measurement. *Small Group Research, 30*(5), 558-581. https://doi.org/10.1177/104649649903000504

Hofstede, G., Neuijen, B., Ohayv, D. D., & Sanders, G. (1990). Measuring Organizational Cultures: A Qualitative and Quantitative Study Across Twenty Cases. *Administrative Science Quarterly, 35*(2), 286-316. https://doi.org/10.2307/2393392

Hollenbeck, J.R., Ellis, A.P.J., Humphrey, S.E., Garza, A.S, & Ilgen, D.R. (2011). Asymmetry in Structural Adaptation: The Differential Impact of Centralizing Versus Decentralizing Team Decision-Making Structures. *Organ Behav Hum Decis Process, 114*(1), 64-74. https://doi.org/10.1016/j.obhdp.2010.08.003

Jehn, K. A., & Mannix, E. A. (2001). The Dynamic Nature of Conflict: A Longitudinal Study of Intragroup Conflict and Group Performance. *Acad Manage J, 44*(2), 238-251. https://doi.org/10.5465/3069453

Kahn, W. A. (1990). Psychological Conditions of Personal Engagement and Disengagement at Work. *Academy of Management Journal, 33*(4), 692-724. https://doi.org/10.5465/256287

Kent, D., & Granqvist, N. (2020). From Clear Skies to EF5s: How Storm Chasing Teams Stay Engaged with Temporally Uncertain Work. *Academy of Management Proceedings, 2020*, 16715. https://doi.org/10.5465/AMBPP.2020.16715abstract

Lang, J. W. B., Bliese, P. D., & de Voogt, A. (2018). Modeling Consensus Emergence in Groups Using Longitudinal Multilevel Methods. *Personnel Psychology, 71*(2), 255-281. https://doi.org/10.1111/peps.12260

Leach, C.W., van Zomeren, M., Zebel, S., Vliek, M.L., Pennekamp, S.F., Doosje, B., Ouwerkerk, J.W., & Spears, R. (2008). Group-Level Self-Definition and Self-Investment: A Hierarchical (Multicomponent) Model of In-Group Identification. *J Pers Soc Psychol. 95*(1). 144-65. doi: 10.1037/0022-3514.95.1.144. PMID: 18605857

Lewis, K. (2003). Measuring Transactive Memory Systems in the Field: Scale Development and Validation. *J Appl Psychol, 88*(4), 587-604. https://doi.org/10.1037/0021-9010.88.4.587

Martin, R., Guillaume, Y., Thomas, G., Lee, A., & Epitropaki, O. (2016). Leader–Member Exchange (LMX) and Performance: A Meta-Analytic Review. *Personnel Psychology, 69*(1), 67-121. https://doi.org/10.1111/peps.12100

Martin, S. R. (2016). Stories about Values and Valuable Stories: A Field Experiment of the Power of Narratives to Shape Newcomers' Actions. *Academy of Management Journal, 59*(5), 1707-1724. https://doi.org/10.5465/amj.2014.0061

Mathieu, J. E., Heffner, T. S., Goodwin, G. F., Salas, E., & Cannon-Bowers, J. A. (2000). The Influence of Shared Mental Models on Team Process and Performance. *J Appl Psychol, 85*, 273-283. https://doi.org/10.1037/0021-9010.85.2.273

Mathieu, J. E., Tannenbaum, S. I., Kukenberger, M. R., Donsbach, J. S., & Alliger, G. M. (2015). Team Role Experience and Orientation: A Measure and Tests of Construct Validity. *Group & Organization Management, 40*(1), 6-34.

Nembhard, I. M., & Edmondson, A. C. (2006). Making It Safe: The Effects of Leader Inclusiveness and Professional Status on Psychological Safety and Improvement Efforts in Health Care Teams. *Journal of Organizational Behavior, 27*(7), 941-966. https://doi.org/10.1002/job.413

Newman, A., Donohue, R., & Eva, N. (2017). Psychological Safety: A Systematic Review of the Literature. *Human Resource Management Review, 27*(3), 521-535. https://doi.org/10.1016/j.hrmr.2017.01.001

Nyberg, A. J., Moliterno, T. P., Hale, D., & Lepak, D. P. (2014). Resource-Based Perspectives on Unit-Level Human Capital: A Review and Integration. *J Manage, 40*(1), 316-346. https://doi.org/10.1177/0149206312458703

Ostroff, C., Shin, Y., & Kinicki, A. J. (2005). Multiple Perspectives of Congruence: Relationships between Value Congruence and Employee Attitudes. *Journal of Organizational Behavior, 26*(6), 591-623. https://doi.

org/10.1002/job.333

Pieper, J. R., Maltarich, M. A., Nyberg, A. J., Reilly, G., & Ray, C. (2023). Collective Turnover Response Over Time to a Unit-Level Shock. *J Appl Psychol, 108*(6), 1001-1026. https://doi.org/10.1037/apl0001052

Rafferty, A. E., & Griffin, M. A. (2006). Refining Individualized Consideration: Distinguishing Developmental Leadership and Supportive Leadership. *Journal of Occupational and Organizational Psychology, 79*(1), 37-61. https://doi.org/10.1348/096317905X36731

Rahim, M. A. (1983). A Measure of Styles of Handling Interpersonal Conflict. *Acad Manage J 26*(2), 368-376. https://doi.org/10.2307/255985

Reilly, G., Nyberg, A. J., Maltarich, M., & Weller, I. (2014). Human Capital Flows: Using Context-Emergent Turnover (CET) Theory to Explore the Process by Which Turnover, Hiring, and Job Demands Affect Patient Satisfaction. *Academy of Management Journal, 57*(3), 766-790. https://doi.org/10.5465/amj.2012.0132

Rossiter, J. R., & Lilien, G. L. (1994). New "Brainstorming" Principles. *Australian Journal of Management, 19*(1), 61-72. https://doi.org/10.1177/031289629401900104

Schweiger, D. M., Sandberg, W. R., & Rechner, P. L. (1989). Experiential Effects of Dialectical Inquiry, Devil's Advocacy, and Consensus Approaches to Strategic Decision Making. *Academy of Management Journal, 32*, 745-772. https://doi.org/10.2307/256567

Schwenk, C. R. (1990). Effects of Devil's Advocacy and Dialectical Inquiry on Decision Making: A Meta-Analysis. *Organizational Behavior and Human Decision Processes, 47*(1), 161-176. https://doi.org/10.1016/0749-5978(90)90051-A

Seashore, S.E. (1954). *Group Cohesiveness in the Industrial Work Group*. University of Michigan Press, Ann Arbor, MI

Sexton, K., Johnson, A., Gotsch, A., Hussein, A. A., Cavuoto, L., & Guru, K. A. (2018). Anticipation, Teamwork and Cognitive Load: Chasing Efficiency during Robot-Assisted Surgery. *BMJ Qual Saf 27*(2), 148. https://doi.org/10.1136/bmjqs-2017-006701

Smith-Jentsch, K. A., Mathieu, J. E., & Kraiger, K. (2005). Investigating Linear and Interactive Effects of Shared Mental Models on Safety and Efficiency in a Field Setting. *J Appl Psychol, 90*(3), 523-535. https://doi.org/10.1037/0021-9010.90.3.523

Stachowski, A. A., Kaplan, S. A., & Waller, M. J. (2009). The Benefits of Flexible Team Interaction during Crises. *J Appl Psychol, 94*(6), 1536-1543. https://doi.org/10.1037/a0016903

Stevens-Haas, C. (2021). Resident reflections early in the COVID19 pandemic: Fear, hope and everything in between. Alliance for Academic Internal Medicine National Meeting, Virtual.

van Zomeren, M., Leach, C. W., & Spears, R. (2010). Does Group Efficacy Increase Group Identification? Resolving their Paradoxical Relationship. *Journal of Experimental Social Psychology, 46*(6), 1055-1060. https://doi.org/10.1016/j.jesp.2010.05.006

Wang, G., Oh, I.-S., Courtright, S. H., & Colbert, A. E. (2011). Transformational Leadership and Performance Across Criteria and Levels: A Meta-Analytic Review of 25 Years of Research. *Group & Organization Management, 36*(2), 223-270. https://doi.org/10.1177/1059601111401017

Zhu J., Liao Z., Yam K.C., & Johnson R.E. (2018). Shared leadership: A State-of-the-Art Review and Future Research Agenda. *J Organ Behav. 39*, 834-852. https://doi.org/10.1002/job.2296

CHAPTER 3

Leading Through a Mental Health Crisis of an Individual Resident

Kathlyn E. Fletcher, MD, MA

Mara Pheister, MD

Medical College of Wisconsin

In this chapter, the authors share two stories of resident mental health crises: a suicidal resident and a resident with a substance use disorder. The stories represent amalgamations of several incidents, and the details have been changed significantly. The stories describe the importance of recognizing the signs that a resident is struggling, using empathic listening, involving others on the leadership team, and having the courage for difficult conversations. Teams with cohesiveness and trust help the program director manage these crises with less stress and isolation.

Introduction

The well-being of physicians, especially residents, has received increasing attention over the last two decades (Baker & Sen, 2016; Dyrbye et al., 2015). Initially, this was related to the relationship between resident burnout and suboptimal patient care (Shanafelt et al., 2002), but resident mental health is important for the residents themselves.

The mental health of Americans overall has declined since the onset of the pandemic (Kaiser Family Foundation). In a 2021 study, 31% of adult Americans report depressive symptoms and/or anxiety, up from 11% before the pandemic (Kaiser Family Foundation). Even before the pandemic, residents/fellows reported significantly higher rates of depression, burnout, fatigue, and low quality of life than their nonresident/fellow peers of similar age (Dyrbye, West, et al., 2014). Poor mental health often begins before residency; approximately 27% of medical students screen positive for depression or depressive symptoms (Rotenstein et al., 2016). Similar numbers of residents screen positive for depression, with rates increasing during residency (Mata et al., 2015). Additionally, women residents develop depression at higher rates than their male counterparts, and work-family conflict may play a role (Guille et al., 2017).

Approximately 4.5% of female and 4.1% of male US adults experienced suicidal ideation between 2015 and 2019. The numbers are higher in the 18-to-39-year-old group, with 6.9% experiencing suicidal ideation (Ivey-Stephenson et al., 2022). While suicidal ideation was just as likely in medical students and residents/fellows as in nonmedical peers (Dyrbye et al., 2015), interns who enter residency with a history of depression or suicidal ideation are at vastly increased risk of having suicidal ideation during their internship (Malone et al., 2021).

Experiencing an increase in work hours and being part of a medical error are also associated with suicidal ideation (Malone et al., 2021). Suicidal ideation is thought to be the result of unbearable psychological pain and hopelessness. While most individuals with suicidal ideation will never make an attempt (Klonsky et al., 2021), suicide is the second leading cause of death among residents and the leading cause of death among male residents (Yaghmour et al., 2017).

Beyond the apparent contribution of residency to anxiety, burnout, and depression, other serious mental illnesses such as schizophrenia, bipolar disorder, and substance use are more common in this age group (National Institute of Mental Health, 2023).

In 2010, Dyrbye and colleagues developed the Physician Well-Being Index (PWBI) to assess well-being in medical students (Dyrbye et al., 2011; Dyrbye et al., 2010). They have since validated it in residents (Dyrbye, Satele, et al., 2014). Low scores on the PWBI are correlated with important resident states such as high fatigue, low mental quality of life, and recent suicidal ideation (Dyrbye, Satele, et al., 2014). In 2021, the PWBI website reported that 17% of resident/fellow physicians were at high risk for distress based on more than 17,000 assessments. Those most at risk were female, second-year residents, and obstetrics/gynecology residents (Well-Being Index, 2022), for unknown reasons.

The Accreditation Council for Graduate Medical Education (ACGME) recognizes the importance of resident well-being and both institutional and programmatic responsibility for promoting well-being through core program requirements (Accreditation Council for Graduate Medical Education, 2022). However, despite the increased emphasis on well-being, some residents still struggle. Given the demographics of the average resident, the national trends in mental health, and the suboptimal levels of well-being during medical training, most program directors will encounter a mental health crisis in a resident.

Story #1: A Resident with Suicidal Ideation

It was a busy early spring afternoon in Wisconsin; it was 38 degrees and overcast. I had a to-do list for the day that was not going to be completed, even if I brought my most-efficient self to the table. I waffled between starting the easiest task (so that I could check something off the list) and the most pressing task (so that I could stop the constant countdown until it was due). I sighed and started the easiest one; I needed a victory.

Five minutes into signing resident verification forms, my pager went off with a message from a chief resident. He wanted to tell me about a resident. He had called Kim (not the resident's real name), a second-year resident, to tell her about an error in the schedule for the upcoming weekend. She was on the Transplant team, which only had two residents, so one of them was always there during the day. The schedule had mistakenly said that Kim had the whole weekend off, but, in fact, she only had Saturday off. Months ago, her co-resident had requested Sunday off to attend his niece's baptism. The chief resident had assured Kim that she would get an additional day off, but it wouldn't be Sunday. This was a disappointing surprise for Kim, and her response to the chief resident delivering this news was rather unprofessional. When he responded by labeling her reaction as "unprofessional," Kim began to cry. Hence, the page to me.

I asked the chief resident to have her come to my office. As I waited, I considered the situation as I knew it. Her reaction seemed extreme, but I didn't know her side of the story. I knew that this part of second year was typically a slog. They are barely half-finished with residency, and it is still months away from delightful weather. "Residency is hard," I thought.

When Kim arrived at my office, I asked her to tell me what was going on from her point of view. She told me that her mother had moved to Wisconsin to be closer to her during residency. About four months ago, her mother was diagnosed with stage 4 ovarian cancer and was now undergoing chemotherapy with an experimental drug. Her mother was having terrible nausea for days after each round of chemotherapy. An only child, Kim bore significant responsibility for taking care of her mother during the cancer treatment and frequently stayed at her mother's apartment after her treatments. Kim told me that she had not been sleeping well since her mother's diagnosis. "There's not enough coffee in the world to overcome this fatigue."

She paused after this disclosure about her mother (which I had not known), and I asked, "What else is happening?" to make sure I had a full understanding of what Kim was facing, not because I had a sense that she was holding back (although I wish that I could claim that level of insight). Kim hesitated and then told me about a difficult patient interaction from months ago that still haunted her. Despite Kim's best efforts to accommodate the substantial emotional and medical needs of the patient and the many requests for updates from the patient's family, she received a formal written complaint from a nurse that the patient's family did not feel that the team, and Kim specifically, were executing the plan that they had expected. The report from the nurse was scathing and had been sent to the hospital's patient advocate, who in turn sent it directly to Kim, asking for a written response within five business days. Kim felt blindsided by the complaint and stunned to see her name listed as a doctor that was providing suboptimal care. She was still hurt from that episode and had not shared it with anyone except the team's attending. I listened and spent some time trying to help her process the interaction. At this point, validating her feelings and experience was the most that I could offer. We talked about how hard it is to take care of patients who are afraid, in pain, and/or very ill.

She started to cry. "I have been thinking about killing myself." But instead of pausing, she immediately began to talk about the scheduling mistake and why Sunday was an important day off for her. I let her continue to talk for a few minutes, but I knew that I would have to backtrack to the suicidal ideation. At the next break in the conversation, I said, "I want to go back to something you said a minute ago about wanting to kill yourself . . . how much have you thought about it? Do you have a plan?"
"I have access to a lot of pills . . . at my mom's house."
We stared at each other. She continued, "It would be painless . . ."

If I am honest, my immediate reaction to this admission was panic (perhaps not the ideal reaction, but it did indicate an understanding that a crisis had begun). I realized that none of the other *things on my to-do list that day were going to happen. I was only going to take care of Kim and her crisis today. That realization was freeing in a way because my whole day had suddenly been cleared to take care of one thing. What should I do? What resources did I have?*

The first priority was to make sure that Kim was safe, but I didn't trust myself to do that alone. One institutional resource available to me was a robust resident mental health program. While the initial attempt to engage that program resulted in us being asked to leave a message or call the emergency department, we quickly pivoted to directly reaching out to the psychologist leader of the resident mental health program. I stepped out of my office while he talked with Kim on the phone. When they finished talking, he talked with me briefly. He told me that she was safe to go home, and that she could be fast-tracked into an appointment with their group.

I had her take the rest of the week/weekend off. I told her that we would arrange coverage, and reminded her that we have a system in place for emergency absences. I checked in with her daily via text/phone over the weekend. We met in person on the following Tuesday. Kim felt much better with some rest and time away from work. We talked through her mother's situation again and decided that a short leave of absence to care for her mother was the best plan.

After her leave of absence, she returned to my office to give me an update. She now had a regular mental health provider and had been able to recruit an aunt and uncle to help care for her mother during the days after her chemotherapy. Her mother had had enough of a response to chemotherapy that she would be able to undergo surgery for resection of the remainder of the tumor. Kim's outlook was much more positive, and she said that she was grateful for the support of the program. I shared some ideas about changes in the program that I was considering because of what I had learned from our interaction, which made her happy. She resumed residency and successfully completed training with her peers.

Advice from the Literature and Practical Wisdom
Recognize that a change in resident behavior may be an important red flag

Mental health, physical health, and other stressors likely influence resident performance (Mitchell et al., 2005; Seehusen, 2020). As in Kim's case, we have seen mental health problems and/or high levels of stress masquerade as "unprofessional" behavior. We always try to explore mental health or stress issues first in conversations with residents about "professionalism problems." "Tell me what happened from your point of view" and "How are you really?" are two possible (and not mutually exclusive) questions that you might use to open your conversation.

Be proactive about patient events involving residents

One study of residents' self-reported errors suggests a two-way relationship between errors and mental health. Committing an error leads to worsening mental health which, in turn, increases the risk of error (West et al., 2006). We also know that burnout appears to have a relationship with self-reported errors (Menon et al., 2020). Therefore, we should proactively address patient care errors and give space for residents to process them. It is not clear if patient complaints are likewise related to resident burnout and mental health, but experience suggests that they can be.

Two possible interventions in the pre-crisis phase include Balint groups (Nalan & Manning, 2022; The American Balint Society, 2024) and Schwartz rounds (Lown & Manning, 2010; The Schwartz Center, 2022). Creating a culture in which teammates debrief with each other when patient care is difficult or when an actual error occurs is invaluable. Having a shared mental model about the importance of such discussions within the leadership group is necessary; spreading it to the core faculty and beyond is the goal. When attending case conferences, the program leadership and core faculty can be mindful of opportunities to call out moments in which the patient case being presented was likely to have been stressful, sad, or difficult. Morbidity and Mortality conferences can specifically include an opportunity to imagine how the team taking care of the patient may have felt as the case was unfolding. Given that these conferences usually involve a suboptimal outcome, spend time identifying the systems factors that contributed rather than focusing on documentation deficiencies or the individual decisions of the doctors ("Medical Errors: Focusing More on What and Why, Less on Who," 2007). Save time to talk about the emotional impact on the team to help the residents (and anyone else attending) process these moments (Berlin & Fletcher, 2021).

The program director or faculty member who is bearing witness to the aftermath, as in this scenario, will need to focus their empathy and listening skills on the learner who is hurting. Normalizing these incidents, emphasizing systems issues that come into play to allow errors to occur, and introducing self-forgiveness are all options in that moment. Being a doctor means taking care of patients on their worst days, and that will always be difficult. With the right support, it can still be meaningful.

Be on the lookout for family and other personal stressors for the residents

Although it hasn't been specifically studied in residents, we know from the literature that major negative life events are correlated with burnout in medical students (Dyrbye et al., 2006). The life events that residents face are what one would expect, based on their age and life stage. You will see breakups and divorces; illnesses and deaths of parents, grandparents, siblings, significant others; and residents' own illnesses and injuries. There is often guilt mixed in with the grief because of the time, energy, and attention that the resident has been devoting to their training leading up to the incident. Sometimes you will hear about these stressors from other residents (or chief residents) who were told the information in confidence. If the resident comes to your attention because a colleague is worried, it can be difficult to directly reach out to the resident in need.

In that case, I will often strategize with the colleague who brought the concern forward. Sometimes they realize that it is okay for the resident in need to know who raised the concern. If they do not want the resident in need to know who brought the concern forward, then work with your team to decide who will approach the resident and what the "reason" is that you reached out to them. Often, I ask the associate program director who knows them best to have the first conversation with them, and we use a generic reason like "some friends are concerned about you; you haven't been yourself lately." Most often, residents are grateful that someone noticed, and it doesn't take long for them to open up about what is happening.

Know your resources

This type of moment is difficult to plan for because you rarely know that it's coming until it is in front of you. The Chapter 1 framework suggests that you would quickly need to assess this situation as the beginning of a crisis and adjust your mindset accordingly.

The first assessment, that of resources, may require you to look outside your immediate leadership team to the resources of your institution. First, remember that you are capable of taking care of this situation. Despite the anxiety you may feel about where this situation could end, you are the right person for this moment; if you weren't, this resident would not be in your office asking for help. Take courage from that knowledge.

The conceptual framework (Chapter 1) helps me think through the next steps logically. I needed the leadership team to enact the relevant processes: communication and coordination. When I knew that Kim needed to take some time off, I asked the chief residents to find coverage for her clinical work. Because I needed to protect her privacy, I could not tell the chief residents the details of what was happening. This is where trust within the team and a shared mental model of how we treat residents who are in crisis are very helpful. The chief residents found coverage immediately without a detailed explanation for why.

I was able to directly engage the director of the resident mental health program. Assessing the risk of suicide in another person is not something that everyone feels comfortable doing. Realistically, unless you are a psychiatrist or a psychologist, you will probably not be in this situation often enough to make it comfortable. Knowing the mental health resources for the residents at your institution is, therefore, a must. I suggest trying to access them on a trial basis. Realizing in the moment of crisis that the mental health emergency number simply goes to the emergency department was very stressful.

When Kim admitted to being suicidal, I was worried that she would refuse to access mental health resources. One aspect of this scenario that may have reduced the barriers is that in the pre-crisis phase, our program leadership discusses the resident mental health resources constantly. If this had been the first time that Kim had heard of them, it might have been harder to convince her to engage with them.

I was fortunate to have easy access to mental health resources, but I recognize that that is not the case for everyone. Regardless of your internal institutional resources, everyone should have access to the suicide crisis line (988) and to an emergency department. Consider how you would manage this as an internal medicine physician if this were a resident having chest pain in front of you. You would do the immediate things first and then have them assessed for a higher level of care. Approach suicidal ideation the same way. Focus on immediate safety first—how intense are the thoughts, is there a plan, do they have access to weapons, what stopped them from acting, and is there someone they can reach out to?

You know to do this because you're a physician, but keep in mind that you are this person's program director, not their doctor. It can be difficult to move between roles sometimes, though speaking as a psychiatrist, I (MP) suspect that this may be a greater risk for our specialty, in particular. Once you've assessed immediate safety, refer and guide them to resources (QPR Institute). You can tell them that you're worried about them and see if they're willing to go to the emergency room. You can call 988 for support or advice. The main thing is enlisting their cooperation to get additional help. Since you've already empathically listened, validated, put all else aside for now, and had them open up to you, you're almost there.

Use leaves of absence liberally

If residents are struggling with life events, taking a leave of absence (LOA) is often the best option. This can range from an extra day off to process the event to a formal leave of absence, maybe using the Family Medical Leave Act (FMLA). Common resident concerns about taking a LOA include worry about graduating late, the impact on future careers, and extra work for their colleagues (Dyrbye et al., 2021).

You can reassure your residents that taking time off to address their mental health needs may not have the long-term repercussions that they imagine. In July 2021, the American Board of Medical Specialties (ABMS) updated its leave policy to allow for more liberal use of LOAs without requiring an extension of training (American Board of Medical Specialties, 2021). If residents remain in training (while on leave), loan deferment will not change. If training does need to be extended, some fellowships will accept fellows off-cycle. If applying for jobs after residency, a later start date would be unlikely to impact their job prospects. That said, extending training for residents with specific situations (National Health Service Corp, certain visa types, military) may be more complicated to navigate.

Residents may be concerned that getting mental health care will affect their ability to be licensed in the future (Aaronson et al., 2018). In 2018, the Federation of State Medical Boards (FSMB) recommended that medical licensure applications and renewals be adapted to focus on current physician impairment, rather than a history of diagnosis or treatment (Federation of State Medical Boards, 2018). A review in 2021 found that while only one state complies with all four evaluable FSMB recommendations, a significant majority of states (72%) used language asking only about physician impairment rather than diagnosis or treatment (Saddawi-Konefka et al., 2021). In my experience as a practicing psychiatrist and program director of 13 years, seeking treatment is not what interferes with careers. Rather, it tends to be the behaviors related to NOT seeking treatment that lead to professional difficulties.

With respect to the extra work for their peers, firmly assure them that they will someday be able to "pay it forward." The good news is that recovery from burnout in medical students is associated with a decrease in suicidal ideation (Dyrbye et al., 2008).

Story #2: Concern for Substance Use

One morning in the late summer, Alex (not the resident's real name) came to my attention because of unusual behavior. His co-residents noted that he would disappear from the team room for hours at a time without explanation. Supervising faculty reported that he was not completing notes for patient encounters. He had also called in sick three times in the last month.

I talked first with the chief residents because I trust them, and they were the ones who told me about some of the behavior changes. When I interviewed the chiefs for the position of chief resident, we developed a shared mental model of how they should talk with struggling residents. Accordingly, the chiefs started by ascertaining the resident's well-being and safety. Next, they got the resident's side of the story. They listened without judgment to Alex's explanations. The chief residents determined that the resident was safe, but a little overwhelmed with the clinical work. They discussed some strategies for completing notes and reminded him of the importance of being available in the team room or communicating if he had to be away, including how to get in touch with him. They planned to follow up with him in a week.

A month later, Alex missed work again. The next day, two residents confidentially told one of the chief residents that Alex was engaging in problematic alcohol use outside of work; they thought that the alcohol use had contributed to his absences.

The APD assigned to track Alex's progress over time met with him. She reviewed his recent absences with him and noted that his teammates had reported that he was sometimes hard to find when he was on duty. She then expressed concern about him and asked to hear his side of the story. "We are worried about you. What is going on?" Alex apologized without offering an explanation. The APD asked him about his alcohol use, and he said that he did use alcohol socially but not to excess. The APD stepped out and called me for advice on next steps.

This was a situation that I had not yet encountered in my time as PD, and I needed some guidance. I reached out to a representative from our graduate medical education office to determine the best way to move forward. Together, we agreed that because of the concerns for active substance use and possible patient safety implications, the best course of action was to put Alex on administrative leave, pending a fitness for duty evaluation. I wanted to speak with him personally first. Before I left my office, I outlined what I wanted to cover at the meeting.

It was an intense meeting. We entered the APD's office. Alex appeared distracted and anxious. We sat down, and I reiterated our concern for his well-being. I asked him to tell me about what had been going on lately. He could not elaborate on anything that was going poorly. I asked him why he thought others might be concerned about him. He did not have any insight. I asked him if he drank alcohol or used any substances. He said that he drank, but not to excess, and that he did not use any other drugs. He was adamant about that. I told him that colleagues were worried that he was drinking more than in the past. He again denied that.

I told him that because of the pattern (recent change in behavior, absences and colleagues' concerns), he would have to be on administrative leave and have a fitness for duty evaluation before he returned to work. Afterward, we alerted our Clinical Competency Committee (CCC) of the situation in case formal remediation or probation was required upon his return. After the fitness for duty examination, he was on administrative leave for seven weeks while he received treatment. Fitness for duty evaluations are confidential; all we know for certain is that he required a medical leave of absence for treatment.

Advice from the Literature and Practical Wisdom

When we consider the conceptual framework, the concept of "fuzzy transitions" is relevant in this case. Are we at the beginning of a crisis when we get the initial report about his behavior, or are we missing important information? At this potential point of equilibrium between pre-crisis and crisis, you should assess trust, shared mental models, deep organizational knowledge, and psychological safety in your leadership team. Managing a situation like this alone is overwhelming, so use your team.

When your leadership team has a shared mental model, individual members will be able to make many decisions without your input. In this case, the chief residents made the decision to take the first steps of informal remediation themselves because of our shared mental model of how to approach these situations.

Unlike the previous scenario, in this case, you have time to anticipate the conversation that you are about to have. Anticipating these conversations can cause anxiety. Anxiety may result in unhelpful emotions such as dread and fear, which can lead to avoidance (Brown, 2021). This is definitely true for me. Because timeliness is crucial in having these conversations, I find it helpful to have a strategy. Here are a few things for you to consider.

Recognize that it takes courage to have these conversations

Just like naming emotions takes some of their power away, I think that naming the character trait that will help me overcome the emotion gives me power. It takes courage to have these conversations.

Be open to hearing their side of the story

This is especially important early on when you are trying to piece together what is really happening. As in the case with the suicidal resident, approach this with curiosity and empathy. While it feels like a crisis for you and your team, it's even more of a crisis for the resident. Validate their feelings and empathize. With that said, your role is not as their confidant or their physician but as their program director. In that role, the only immediate decision you are making is whether this person will return to work after this meeting. You do not need to determine the extent of their illness or interrogate them. Hear them, help them reach out for support, and let them know when you will talk next.

Plan your conversation

As mentioned above, use your leadership team—they have ideas, help, and support to offer. If your APDs and/or program coordinator have deep organizational knowledge of the institution and faculty, they may be able to advise you on contingencies that you had not anticipated. If your leadership team has psychological safety, then the others on your leadership team can offer perspectives and recommendations that are different from yours without the fear that their standing on the team will be at risk. Involving your leadership team formally or informally (as time allows) will remind you why these conversations are necessary and may give you a different perspective on how to approach the situation.

Outline the conversation ahead of time

Write down the points that you know you need to make. For example, I always start with a statement about my personal concern for the person I am meeting. If you are struggling with how to phrase some part of the message that you have to deliver, write the entire sentence out. Writing it out may keep you from sugarcoating the message in the actual moment. If there are specific things you have to say because of institutional policies surrounding the issue, then write the entire sentence. For example, instead of writing "fitness for duty examination," I write "In order for us to understand what is happening, you will need to have a fitness for duty examination." These conversations require honesty. The honesty doesn't have to be brutal, but it does have to be clear. This is the time to use radical candor, a concept that combines caring about the resident and being completely honest at the same time (Scott, 2017). I actually take the notecard with my outline into the meeting with me. That way, I do not have the additional stress of worrying that my mind might go blank.

Prepare yourself ahead of time as you might mentally prepare for a potentially contentious family meeting in the ICU. Recognize that you will have heightened emotions (dread, fear, anger, guilt, annoyance, among others). Take a few moments to acknowledge this and to center yourself.

Have another person in the room
Because these meetings can turn contentious, and it is hard to remember everything that you say and that the resident says, having another person present (e.g., an APD) can be immensely helpful. This is also a trust-building opportunity if you ask for the APD's critique of the meeting afterward. You could also consider having a chief resident present to support the resident during and after the meeting. You should give the resident the choice of having the chief resident there because confidentiality may be more important than support to the resident.

Room for Improvement
The other residents want an update that you cannot provide
This is a real communication problem that occurs when a resident is struggling. It is not specific to substance use. Not saying anything is not the right answer, which we learned from experience. Having a resident in your program who is struggling is usually noticed by the other residents. Sometimes they have provided personal support to that resident. Sometimes they have observed unsafe or suboptimal patient care from that resident. Even if the program has intervened, the other residents may assume that your leadership group is not taking appropriate action. Our experience is that the other residents will usually go to the chief residents with these complaints. The chiefs will need your help in crafting an appropriate message such as this: "We wouldn't disclose information about you to your peers, so please do not assume that just because you are not aware of any actions about your colleague that no actions are being taken."

Be appropriately suspicious

It is human nature to give people the benefit of the doubt, as described in Malcolm Gladwell's book Talking to Strangers (Gladwell, 2019). In several cases of substance use disorder, we missed early signs in residents that seem obvious now. The behaviors were consistent with the diagnosis, but the residents had reasonable other explanations, and we wanted to believe them. Sometimes their explanations were outright falsehoods. Diagnosis and treatment delays occurred. Luckily, patients were not harmed, but they could have been. Listen to the suspicious voice in your head. Get input from the CCC and your leadership team. Use kindness and empathy but also firmness and resolve. If your suspicion is based on signs that are consistent with substance use disorder, refer them for a fitness for duty examination.

Summary

Cases of mental health crises in residents are not rare. You may not have warning that they are evolving. Building team attributes such as trust, shared mental models, deep organizational knowledge, and psychological safety pay off when these situations occur. Courage, empathy, and honesty are required. Anticipate the difficulty of communicating a message to the entire program without providing them the details that they want to hear.

Table 1. Summary approach to residents with possible serious mental illness	
Pre-Crisis	Establish shared mental models with APDs and chief residents; allow them to have the initial conversation with the resident Monitor the transition: Is this a crisis?

Crisis	Assess the safety of the resident (and the patients)
	    Is it possible that a resident is impaired and that is affecting patient care?
	    Is the resident suicidal?
	Get the resident's side of the story
	Use empathic listening
	Enlist your team's help for planning and support
	Implement a plan and alert/engage the CCC

Post-Crisis	Communicate with the other residents (if indicated)

Citations

Aaronson, A. L., Backes, K., Agarwal, G., Goldstein, J. L., & Anzia, J. (2018). Mental Health During Residency Training: Assessing the Barriers to Seeking Care. *Acad Psychiatry, 42*(4), 469-472. https://doi.org/10.1007/s40596-017-0881-3

Accreditation Council for Graduate Medical Education. (2022). *ACGME - Common Program Requirements (Residency)*. https://www.acgme.org/globalassets/PFAssets/ProgramRequirements/CPRResidency_2022v2.pdf

American Board of Medical Specialties. (2021). *American Board of Medical Specialties Policy on Parental, Caregiver and Medical Leave During Training*. American Board of Medical Specialties. Retrieved May 23, 2023 from https://www.abms.org/policies/parental-leave/

Baker, K., & Sen, S. (2016). Healing Medicine's Future: Prioritizing Physician Trainee Mental Health. *AMA J Ethics, 18*(6), 604-613. https://doi.org/10.1001/journalofethics.2016.18.6.medu1-1606

Berlin K, & Fletcher K. (2021). Mini M&M Conferences Create a Structured Opportunity for Self-Reflection. National American College of Physicians Meeting.

Brown, B. (2021). *Atlas of the Heart: Mapping Meaningful Connection and the Language of Human Experience* (First edition ed.). Random House, New York.

Dyrbye, L. N., Eacker, A., Durning, S. J., Brazeau, C., Moutier, C., Massie, F. S., Satele, D., Sloan, J. A., & Shanafelt, T. D. (2015). The Impact of Stigma and Personal Experiences on the Help-Seeking Behaviors of Medical Students With Burnout. *Acad Med, 90*(7), 961-969. https://doi.org/10.1097/acm.0000000000000655

Dyrbye, L. N., Leep Hunderfund, A. N., Winters, R. C., Moeschler, S. M., Vaa Stelling, B. E., Dozois, E. J., Satele, D. V., & West, C. P. (2021). The Relationship Between Burnout and Help-Seeking Behaviors, Concerns, and Attitudes of Residents. *Acad Med, 96*(5), 701-708. https://doi.org/10.1097/acm.0000000000003790

Dyrbye, L. N., Satele, D., Sloan, J., & Shanafelt, T. D. (2014). Ability of the Physician Well-Being Index to Identify Residents in Distress. *J Grad Med Educ, 6*(1), 78-84. https://doi.org/10.4300/jgme-d-13-00117.1

Dyrbye, L. N., Schwartz, A., Downing, S. M., Szydlo, D. W., Sloan, J. A., & Shanafelt, T. D. (2011). Efficacy of a Brief Screening Tool to Identify Medical Students in Distress. *Acad Med, 86*(7), 907-914. https://doi.org/10.1097/ACM.0b013e31821da615

Dyrbye, L. N., Szydlo, D. W., Downing, S. M., Sloan, J. A., & Shanafelt, T. D. (2010). Development and Preliminary Psychometric Properties of a Well-Being Index for Medical Students. *BMC Med Educ, 10*, 8. https://doi.org/10.1186/1472-6920-10-8

Dyrbye, L. N., Thomas, M. R., Huntington, J. L., Lawson, K. L., Novotny, P. J., Sloan, J. A., & Shanafelt, T. D. (2006). Personal Life Events and Medical Student Burnout: A Multicenter Study. *Acad Med, 81*(4), 374-384. https://doi.org/10.1097/00001888-200604000-00010

Dyrbye, L. N., Thomas, M. R., Massie, F. S., Power, D. V., Eacker, A., Harper, W., Durning, S., Moutier, C., Szydlo, D. W., Novotny, P. J., Sloan, J. A., & Shanafelt, T. D. (2008). Burnout and Suicidal Ideation among U.S. Medical Students. *Ann Intern Med, 149*(5), 334-341. https://doi.org/10.7326/0003-4819-149-5-200809020-00008

Dyrbye, L. N., West, C. P., Satele, D., Boone, S., Tan, L., Sloan, J., & Shanafelt, T. D. (2014). Burnout among U.S. Medical Students, Residents, and Early Career Physicians Relative to the General U.S. Population. *Acad Med, 89*(3), 443-451. https://doi.org/10.1097/acm.0000000000000134

Federation of State Medical Boards. (2018). *Physician Wellness and Burnout: Report and Recommendations of the Workgroup on Physician Wellness and Burnout*. https://www.fsmb.org/siteassets/advocacy/policies/policy-on-wellness-and-burnout.pdf

Gladwell, M. (2019). *Talking to Strangers: What We Should Know about the People We Don't Know*. Little, Brown, and Company.

Guille, C., Frank, E., Zhao, Z., Kalmbach, D. A., Nietert, P. J., Mata, D. A., & Sen, S. (2017). Work-Family Conflict and the Sex Difference in Depression Among Training Physicians. *JAMA Intern Med, 177*(12), 1766-1772. https://doi.org/10.1001/jamainternmed.2017.5138

Ivey-Stephenson, A. Z., Crosby, A. E., Hoenig, J. M., Gyawali, S., Park-Lee, E., & Hedden, S. L. (2022). Suicidal Thoughts and Behaviors Among Adults Aged ≥18 Years - United States, 2015-2019. *MMWR Surveill Summ, 71*(1), 1-19. https://doi.org/10.15585/mmwr.ss7101a1

Kaiser Family Foundation. (December 13, 2021). *Mental Health and Substance Use State Fact Sheets*. Kaiser Family Foundation. Retrieved December 20, 2022 from https://www.kff.org/interactive/mental-health-and-substance-use-state-fact-sheets/

Klonsky, E. D., Dixon-Luinenburg, T., & May, A. M. (2021). The Critical Distinction between Suicidal Ideation and Suicide Attempts. *World Psychiatry, 20*(3), 439-441. https://doi.org/10.1002/wps.20909

Lown, B. A., & Manning, C. F. (2010). The Schwartz Center Rounds: Evaluation of an Interdisciplinary Approach to Enhancing Patient-Centered Communication, Teamwork, and Provider Support. *Acad Med, 85*(6), 1073-1081. https://doi.org/10.1097/ACM.0b013e3181dbf741

Malone, T. L., Zhao, Z., Liu, T. Y., Song, P. X. K., Sen, S., & Scott, L. J. (2021). Prediction of Suicidal Ideation Risk in a Prospective Cohort Study of Medical Interns. *PLoS One, 16*(12), e0260620. https://doi.org/10.1371/journal.pone.0260620

Mata, D. A., Ramos, M. A., Bansal, N., Khan, R., Guille, C., Di Angelantonio, E., & Sen, S. (2015). Prevalence of Depression and Depressive Symptoms Among Resident Physicians: A Systematic Review and Meta-Analysis. *Jama, 314*(22), 2373-2383. https://doi.org/10.1001/jama.2015.15845

Medical Errors: Focusing More on What and Why, Less on Who. (2007). *J Oncol Pract, 3*(2), 66-70. https://doi.org/10.1200/jop.0723501

Menon, N. K., Shanafelt, T. D., Sinsky, C. A., Linzer, M., Carlasare, L., Brady, K. J. S., Stillman, M. J., & Trockel, M. T. (2020). Association of Physician Burnout With Suicidal Ideation and Medical Errors. *JAMA Netw Open, 3*(12), e2028780. https://doi.org/10.1001/jamanetworkopen.2020.28780

Mitchell, M., Srinivasan, M., West, D. C., Franks, P., Keenan, C., Henderson, M., & Wilkes, M. (2005). Factors Affecting Resident Performance: Development of a Theoretical Model and a Focused Literature Review. *Acad Med, 80*(4), 376-389. https://doi.org/10.1097/00001888-200504000-00016

Nalan, P., & Manning, A. (2022). The Juice is Worth the Squeeze: Psychiatry Residents' Experience of Balint Group. *Int J Psychiatry Med, 57*(6), 508-520. https://doi.org/10.1177/00912174221127084

National Institute of Mental Health. (2023, March 2023). *Mental Illness Statistics*. National Institute of Health. Retrieved May 23, 2023 from https://www.nimh.nih.gov/health/statistics/mental-illness

QPR Institute. *What is QPR?* QPR Institute. Retrieved May 23, 2023 from https://qprinstitute.com/about-qpr

Rotenstein, L. S., Ramos, M. A., Torre, M., Segal, J. B., Peluso, M. J., Guille, C., Sen, S., & Mata, D. A. (2016). Prevalence of Depression, Depressive Symptoms, and Suicidal Ideation Among Medical Students: A Systematic Review and Meta-Analysis. *JAMA, 316*(21), 2214-2236. https://doi.org/10.1001/jama.2016.17324

Saddawi-Konefka, D., Brown, A., Eisenhart, I., Hicks, K., Barrett, E., & Gold, J. A. (2021). Consistency Between State Medical License Applications and Recommendations Regarding Physician Mental Health. *JAMA, 325*(19), 2017-2018. https://doi.org/10.1001/jama.2021.2275

Scott, K. (2017). *Radical Candor: How to be a Kickass Boss without Losing your Humanity* (First edition. ed.). St. Martin's Press.

Seehusen, D. A. (2020). Understanding Unprofessionalism in Residents. *J Grad Med Educ, 12*(3), 243-246. https://doi.org/10.4300/jgme-d-19-00668.1

Shanafelt, T. D., Bradley, K. A., Wipf, J. E., & Back, A. L. (2002). Burnout and Self-Reported Patient Care in an Internal Medicine Residency Program. *Ann Intern Med, 136*(5), 358-367. https://doi.org/10.7326/0003-4819-136-5-200203050-00008

The American Balint Society. (2024). *What is a Balint Group?* Retrieved January 24, 2024 from https://american-balintsociety.org/what_is_a_balint_group.php

The Schwartz Center. (2022). *What We Do.* The Schwartz Center. Retrieved May 5, 2023 from https://www.theschwartzcenter.org/about/what-we-do/

Well-Being Index. (2022). *State of Well-Being 2021-2022.* https://www.mywellbeingindex.org/insights

West, C. P., Huschka, M. M., Novotny, P. J., Sloan, J. A., Kolars, J. C., Habermann, T. M., & Shanafelt, T. D. (2006). Association of Perceived Medical Errors with Resident Distress and Empathy: A Prospective Longitudinal Study. *JAMA, 296*(9), 1071-1078. https://doi.org/10.1001/jama.296.9.1071

Yaghmour, N. A., Brigham, T. P., Richter, T., Miller, R. S., Philibert, I., Baldwin, D. C., Jr., & Nasca, T. J. (2017). Causes of Death of Residents in ACGME-Accredited Programs 2000 Through 2014: Implications for the Learning Environment. *Acad Med, 92*(7), 976-983. https://doi.org/10.1097/acm.0000000000001736

CHAPTER 4

Leading through a Serious Illness and Death of a Resident

Kathlyn E. Fletcher, MD, MA
Medical College of Wisconsin

Jillian Catalanotti, MD, MPH
George Washington University School of Medicine and Health Sciences

Amy S. Oxentenko, MD
Mayo Clinic School of Medicine

In this chapter, the authors describe two resident deaths, one from a prolonged illness and another from suicide. The details have been changed and multiple situations merged to protect the privacy of those involved. These heart-wrenching stories illustrate that PDs need to call on their courage, resilience, and love in the darkest of times to guide their residents, leadership teams, and even the family of the resident that died.

Introduction

Serious illness and/or death of a resident is perhaps the most difficult crisis to experience for program directors. A 2017 paper reported 324 resident deaths in ACGME-accredited residency programs between 2000 and 2014. The most common cause was cancer (26% of deaths in which the cause was determined), with suicide (21%) the second-leading cause (Yaghmour et al., 2017). Regardless of the cause, the death of a resident is devastating. However, there are some differences in leadership approach depending on whether you are facing a resident's serious illness or the death of a resident.

A review of the literature does not offer much guidance for how to lead during times of tragedy such as the serious illness or death of a resident. One firsthand account from a co-resident offers insight into the profound sadness and anxiety that occurs when a "member of the (residency) family" dies (Khan, 2017). When a resident dies, the residents who remain will need you. Program directors must grieve and also allow for the grief of their leadership teams. PDs must also console the residents, family, and others left behind.

Story #1: Death of a Resident Following a Serious Illness

I had only been the program director for three months. The September morning was hot and humid, and I was glad to reach the coolness of my office. As I waited for my computer to update, one of the chief residents approached my office, looking uncharacteristically flustered. "Come in, Ted. What's on your mind?" I said, studying his face. He closed the door and sat in the extra chair across from me.

With a look of dread in his eyes, he took a deep breath and began to tell me his concern for a resident. "Last week, Javi told me that he had been having back pain for weeks. He said he was having a hard time sleeping. And it was thoracic. I was worried when he told me the details, and I helped him get an MRI scheduled. It was done yesterday." He paused, and I was startled as he blinked back tears. "It looks like a metastatic lesion." With that news, the first real crisis of my time as program director began.

A complete workup followed, and Javi elected to have his cancer treated at our medical center. I took stock of Javi's support system. He had a small group of very close friends in the residency program, and he lived with his wife. However, his parents and siblings had moved back to South America before he began his residency training.

I spoke to Javi early on about how he would prefer I talk with the residents and faculty about him, given that he would be away from work and everyone would be worried. He was a private person and laid out his vision clearly. He did not want an email blast sent out, but he was fine with the other residents being given the simple message that he had been diagnosed with cancer, was getting treatment here, and would be away from work for an uncertain amount of time. With respect to the faculty, he only wanted those directly involved in his care to know anything. He wanted the chief residents and me to know everything. Initially, I didn't even share his situation with the associate program directors.

At our institution, we have teaching and non-teaching teams, so the chief residents kept Javi (as a patient) on non-teaching teams for the first year of his illness. During that time, he was able to work intermittently, and we arranged electives for him to complete even when his energy was low and he had to be at home. I personally checked in with him (usually by text or phone) every few weeks. When he was hospitalized, I paid one visit per hospitalization. I remember Javi's humor so distinctly. At one point, he asked me to tell the other residents not to ever order the lemon-lime flavored magnesium citrate for patients because it was "disgusting." He much preferred the cherry flavor, and we joked about that for months. His upbeat nature made it both easier and harder to watch him go through treatment after treatment, each offering at most only small improvements.

Javi was admitted to the hospital late one night almost a year after his diagnosis. The only teams that admit patients after midnight are the resident teams, and so for the first time, he was admitted to a team staffed by our residents. As luck would have it, the senior resident that night, Jenna, was one of Javi's friends. The following morning, Jenna stopped by my office to tell me a story that still brings me to tears.

When she learned of Javi's admission, she reviewed his medical record. She then went to see him. After she completed her assessment, she steeled herself for what she knew she had to say. "Javi, I just finished a rotation on Palliative Care. After reviewing your history, I think that you need to see them." It was the first time anyone had said that to him. He slowly nodded and said that he agreed. As she told me the story, I could see that she was overwhelmed with the responsibility of having to say that to a friend, but she was certain she had done the right thing. I was blown away by her courage and honesty in that moment and hoped I would do the same thing if ever in that position.

That hospital stay marked a turning point for Javi and his journey. The palliative care team, led by one particular faculty member, assumed care of everyone. They treated the residency program as if they were Javi's extended family; they didn't share medical information, but they were fully present to offer support to us all. On one occasion, the palliative faculty leader reached out to me about another resident she was worried about. She had observed a resident from another consult team in Javi's room during a family meeting and could sense the deep sadness and discomfort the resident was feeling. I was able to reach out to this resident and offer comfort and a chance to debrief with me.

Javi decided to stop treatment and move to South America to be with his family for whatever time he had left. During one of my visits with him, Javi told me how much he wished that he could complete the program. I called our designated institutional official (DIO) to ask about how we could still give Javi a certificate of completion before he left. There was more red tape than I had imagined, but finally, we were able to make it happen. We planned a small ceremony with Javi's friends present, and his family made the trip from South America to be there for his "graduation." There were smiles and tears—even laughter—as we celebrated this brave, kind soul and his accomplishments.

A month later, I received a text from Javi's wife that he had died. I walked into the chief residents' office and waited for them to get back from running morning report. They looked at me questioningly as they filed in. I closed the door and started to cry. "Javi is gone." We stood there together, each trying to make sense of his death and trying to find a way through the rest of the day. One of them said, "I know this is a strange thing to say, but I am kind of relieved to see you cry. We had all been wondering how you were holding up, and now we know."

By this time, many of our residents had never worked with Javi, but his classmates were PGY3s. We sent an email letting all residents and faculty know of Javi's passing and reserved a room on campus outside of the hospital for any who wanted to come by after work to share thoughts or stories, or to just be together. Because I didn't have rapid access to mental health providers, our palliative care faculty member graciously agreed to join us to provide support. I wondered what I would say and reviewed Javi's online evaluations, where I quickly discovered his remarkable peer evaluations, stating what a supportive teammate, selfless teacher, and compassionate doctor he was. When his classmates were at first slow to share stories, I shared some evaluation examples, citing how wonderful it was that, through our evaluations, we had already told Javi how very special we all thought he was.

Advice from the Literature and Practical Wisdom

Actively manage privacy issues

Privacy is an issue for program directors in many facets of our work, but resident illness is an especially fraught time. Both faculty and residents will want to know what is happening because they are curious and because they are worried about their colleague. Additionally, some residents will want justification for why they need to cover for someone else. When a resident is facing a diagnosis that will result in a prolonged leave of absence, you will have to actively manage the messaging to faculty and the other residents.

I talked with Javi after his diagnosis to obtain his input about messaging. Having very specific guidance from the resident allows them to have some control in an out-of-control situation. Javi allowed me to share his basic diagnosis with the residents, but he did not want it in an email. I am glad that he was so specific because writing an email to deliver news to the program is almost reflexive. Delivering the news in person was awkward because I did not have permission to provide any additional information when answering follow-up questions. However, being in person gave me a touchpoint with the other residents during a difficult moment, providing some comfort to them.

If a resident does not want any information about their illness shared with the program, ask them for more specific guidance: "What would you like me to say when your co-residents ask me if you are okay?" You could have some ideas to suggest, such as "Javi has asked us not to discuss his absence with anyone right now" or "I know that it is difficult not knowing what is happening with a colleague, but I would respect your wishes for confidentiality if you were in his shoes." Presumably, a resident facing serious illness would not want to field questions from individual colleagues, but maybe they would rather you refer residents with questions directly to them. Regardless, it's helpful to agree on what you and others in your leadership group will say when asked about the absence.

> *"If a resident does not want any information about their illness shared with the program, ask them for more specific guidance: "What would you like me to say when your co-residents ask me if you are okay?"*

Once information is out in the community, it is difficult to control its spread. Because Javi specifically requested not to have his medical information shared with faculty who were not involved in his care, we felt even more protective of his privacy. At one point, I learned of faculty talking about Javi's situation and had to talk with them about his wish for privacy. It was difficult and awkward for me to police that, but I felt responsible. In our situation, recalling Javi's words gave us the courage to be firm in our expectations for maintaining his privacy.

Assign a person to be the primary contact
Having a specific person (or a small group) to check in with the resident who is sick is better for the resident because the continuity saves them the effort of having to provide background information to a new person each time something happens. It may also give them a deeper connection to that person, which could add to their support network. I assigned one chief resident to be the primary contact between Javi and the residency leadership group. As a PD, giving the task of primary contact to a chief resident demonstrated trust of the chiefs and eased my responsibilities as well.

Define your own role in the crisis early
You will need clarity around your personal role in supporting a resident with a serious illness. For example, I decided that I would visit once per hospitalization. Before making this decision, I was torn between wanting to spend time offering direct support and wanting to give him space/time to focus on his treatment. It was also hard on me every time I visited because the situation was just so sad. As doctors, we routinely bear witness to very difficult moments for so many of our patients. It is different when the patient is someone in your own circle; it can be overwhelming and intense. It is hard to turn off the desire to have all the information that the team knows, and yet that is not our role in those moments. Our role is closer to that of a family member, especially in cases like Javi's in which there are so few family members nearby. Having a self-assigned role with parameters was helpful in managing these competing issues and feelings.

Share how you are feeling with your leadership team
As a leader, you may be tempted to project only strength during crisis. Make sure that you allow your feelings to show as well. I did not cry in the presence of my leadership team until the day Javi died. My leadership team had wondered how I was feeling throughout Javi's illness journey, but I did not realize that. For some PDs, showing emotions, especially during a crisis,

may not come naturally. Realize that your team may be looking to you for cues about how to feel or how to share their own feelings. Even if you are not comfortable crying with others, talk about how you are feeling. Showing your own vulnerability will help others in your group who are struggling.

Use peer evaluations when planning a memorial service
Having a memorial service that allows for the attendance of residents, faculty, and staff who knew the resident is imperative. Memorial services are part of the healing process, and the funeral planned by the resident's family may occur in a location too far away for many program colleagues to attend.

When I started planning Javi's memorial service, I was initially at a loss for how to talk about him to a large, diverse audience, some of whom only knew *of* him. The comments from his evaluations, especially his peer evaluations, were a treasure trove of beautiful reflections about the person he was. Reading others' evaluations may make your own statements easier to formulate. I also found that having a few evaluations on hand to share was a good segue into the part of the memorial when I asked other people to share their memories. Additionally, have a few people prepared to share a story.

Room for Improvement
Know your available mental health resources
Assess mental health resources in the pre-crisis phase. I did not know all the mental health resources available to residents when my crisis began. In our situation, the palliative care service filled the role of caring for the whole program. That was outside their scope of practice, but they cared about the other residents and wanted to help. Other options may include faculty (or senior residents) from the Department of Psychiatry. If your site has student/resident mental health services, contact them to inquire about program-wide resources for grief/anxiety. If neither of these options are available to you, ask your chair what financial resources would be available should you need them. One colleague realized that her residents needed space and time to talk about the daily difficulties of residency after a crisis. She asked the Department of Psychiatry at her institution if they knew of anyone available to have regular meetings with the residents. They sent a faculty member once a month for free. It never hurts to ask!

Engage available mental health resources early

As soon as it crosses your mind that you might need mental health resources for your program, you do. It is rarely wrong to make them available to your residents. If your residents have access to individual mental health care, a crisis like this is a good time to remind them that those resources exist. Be pushy. Send the phone number out to the whole group. Anytime you talk with an individual resident, remind them that these resources exist for a reason. Make it easy for them to step away, even during work hours.

Strongly consider using some conference time to have a psychologist or psychiatrist meet with the residents together. As discussed above, a palliative care faculty member could serve in this role, but consider asking for someone who has not been involved with the care of the resident who died. It may be best to not have the program leadership there so that the residents feel like they can speak openly. I know PDs who have tried to lead sessions like this in their programs, and it can result in complete silence. While it is important for the PD to be visible during a crisis, this particular intervention may be best accomplished by a trained outsider. The timing may be complicated because if you are being proactive and engaging mental health resources early, you cannot arrange a session to prepare for the death of a resident. However, you can say that you are scheduling a session because you have noticed an increase in the stress and anxiety in your program. What the residents choose to talk about at the session is not within your control, but at least you have put the resources they need in front of them.

Give chief residents the job of finding residents that are suffering

I wish that I had been more proactive about identifying residents in our program who were suffering during and after Javi's illness. Chief residents are in a much better position than PDs to understand the connections within the program. I did not know who all of Javi's close friends were, and there could have been others not close to him who were disproportionately affected by his illness and death. In the next crisis, I would ask the chief residents to keep their ears to the ground and even ask around about who may be having a hard time. Especially in large programs, it is easy for one resident who is suffering to escape the notice of the leadership group, but someone might know. Demonstrating through the chief residents that we are worried about the survivors could have made it easier for others to seek help if needed or to at least have someone to talk with about their feelings. See the Box in Chapter 5 for suggestions of how to engage in conversations with peers when you are worried about them.

Table 1. Summary approach to the serious illness of a resident	
Pre-Crisis	Know the available mental health resources for the residents
Crisis	Pause and consider the privacy issues
	Assign a primary contact between the resident and the program
	Define your own role
	Engage the mental health resources available to the residents early
	Attend to the emotions of the residents and leadership team
	Share your feelings with the rest of your team
Post-Crisis	Plan a memorial (if indicated)
	Watch for continued grief in the residents

Story #2: A Resident Suicide

"Happy birthday!" I said as my young daughter opened the back door to my car. She was giddy because we were leaving school early for a special birthday lunch at her favorite Thai restaurant. I smiled as we got out of the car and walked into the restaurant hand in hand.

As we sat down and started looking at the menu, my phone pinged with an incoming text. Robin, one of the chief residents, was alerting me that an intern was 30 minutes late to her shift on the general medicine wards, and the chief residents hadn't been able to reach her. We thought it likely that she had overslept, but Robin decided she would go to her apartment to be sure.

After my daughter and I ordered our food, my phone rang, and Robin's number appeared on the screen. I felt prickles of dread on my skin as I answered. "I'm at Annette's apartment," she reported in a panic-tinged voice. "There are police cars and yellow tape everywhere. They won't tell me anything." Her voice cracked. "I don't know what to do." I motioned for the server and told Robin I would meet her back at my office right away. We got our food to go, and I dropped off my daughter back at school as I hurried to my office.

I met with my program coordinator and Robin to try to piece together what had happened. We called the police department and were only told that there was an "investigation" ongoing. After an hour and a half, we received a call from Annette's mother. She, Annette's father, and her high-school-aged brother were on their way to us from South Carolina, a 10-hour drive. Annette had died. They were in shock, but I could hear the unspoken accusation in her mother's voice: This might have been a suicide, and I had missed the signs that she was struggling.

I called the APDs to my office and broke the news to them. I paused, absorbing their silence and grief. "How do we manage the rest of the residents? How do we tell them?" I asked the group. As I looked around the room, I realized that we were almost paralyzed with the emotional weight of the moment. I realized that I was going to have to snap into a different mindset in order to get through the next few hours, so I started delegating tasks. I assigned people to reserve an auditorium, to contact services and clinics so that residents could be freed up for a meeting, and to contact the residents to let them know that there was a mandatory meeting at 4:00 PM. I spent the next several hours talking to departmental, GME, and institutional leadership as well as to our medical-legal department. I barely finished those tasks before I had to go to the auditorium to make one of the hardest announcements of my life.

I told the residents simply that Annette had died and we did not know any details yet. They were stunned, and a few of the other interns started to cry. We had pastoral services and a psychologist at the meeting to offer immediate support. The leadership group stayed to offer comfort to the residents. We asked the PGY3 residents to cover the interns who were scheduled to be in the hospital that night so the interns could be together to process the loss of their colleague.

After the meeting, I waited in my office for Annette's parents and brother to arrive because they wanted to meet with me right away. We still did not know the cause of death at that point, but they articulated their strong suspicion that she had died by suicide. While we were meeting, they received a call from the coroner's office confirming that Annette had overdosed in an apparent suicide.

The meeting with Annette's parents was hard. They were understandably suspicious of why the program had not noticed her struggling. They wondered whether the program was too rigorous. However, they also shared some details about Annette's background that we had not known about, specifically a mental health diagnosis that put her at risk. We talked about what the program could say to the other residents who were already asking what had happened and were certainly forming their own narratives in the absence of actual information. Annette's parents *were not ready for that disclosure, and I wasn't sure if they would ever be. I knew I had to respect their wishes.*

Over the next few months, I met with or talked with Annette's family every few weeks. We talked about her, her life, and her legacy. Slowly, her parents realized that Annette's story could prevent other residents from struggling in silence. Finally, her parents gave consent for me to share her story.

From then on, I shared her story with each new class of interns during orientation. We wanted our interns to know that they were not alone, that we would support them through all kinds of struggles, and that we might not be able to see what was going on in their worlds because they were often so good at hiding it. Annette's story and the message emanating from it have been very powerful forces in our program, and I am still so grateful for her family's courage and humility in letting us share it.

Advice from the Literature and Practical Wisdom

Find your starting point

Determine if your GME office has a policy to enact or an algorithm to follow when an unexpected resident death is discovered. If your institution does not have such a policy, there is an excellent resource available online (Dyrbye et al., 2017) that walks through the management of a resident suicide; many of the steps also could be applied to a non-suicide death. The AFSP checklist is a good place to start.

Table 2. Checklist for After a Suicide - *Printed with permission from AFSP*	
Day 1	Immediate notifications (see Figure 1)* Meeting(s) with residents If not already in place, develop a Crisis Response Team using the template on Page 5*
Day 2	Remaining announcements (see Figure 1)* Check in individually with any at-risk residents Use noon conference to debrief with residents with mental health professional If Chairperson was not at earlier meetings with residents, beginning of this meeting is another opportunity for him/her to check in with residents Check in with deceased resident's emergency contact/family regarding funeral arrangements and next steps, plans to meet

Day 3-4	Consider cancelling didactics and convening residents to gather
	If possible, provide meals over the weekend. Ask attending(s) covering the weekend to check in
	For residents not on call for the weekend encourage informal gatherings
	Let residents and faculty know about funeral arrangements and address for condolence cards/social media site
	Debrief with Crisis Response Team
Week 1	Check in daily with Chief Residents (CRs) – they will be on the frontline and will know who is struggling; this is also a very difficult time for CRs
	Crisis Response Team continues to meet for debrief, monitoring of community, and carry out of communication next steps
Week 2	Return to regularly scheduled didactics
	Make statement that this is still early in grieving process, reinforce continued availability of mental health services, caring for each other, faculty who are available to speak, etc.
	Check in with family regarding any HR issues (benefits, final paycheck, hospital apartment, returning of electronic devices, etc.) and Memorial Service
	Plan Memorial Service
	Ask faculty advisors to check in with advisees, plan group dinners, etc.
	Debrief with the Crisis Response Team
	Provide suicide loss resources to community/appropriate individuals (afsp.org/AfterALoss)
Week 3-4	Consider another noon conference to debrief with residents with mental health professional
	Continue checking in with CRs and think about best ways to support them (take them out for nice lunch or dinner)
	Continue to monitor schedules and work flow
	Monitor residents coping as described above
	Debrief with the Crisis Response Team – refine plan
Beyond the first month	Hold memorial service if not done already
	Consider monthly process groups with mental health professional
	Attend to resident wellbeing issues
	Develop a departmental resident wellbeing plan
	If not already done, develop an institutional suicide prevention plan

*See the AFSP resource website for the Figure and Template. https://www.acgme.org/globalassets/pdfs/13287_afsp_after_suicide_clinician_toolkit_final_2.pdf

The first recommendation is to have a crisis response team. Ideally, a crisis response team is identified in the pre-crisis phase, although depending on the exact nature of the crisis, the leadership of the team may change. For a resident death, the PD will often be the crisis response team leader. The team would likely include the DIO, a mental health resource, and a staff person, among others.

Clear your own schedule of clinical work for at least a week
When such an acute, traumatic event like the loss of a trainee occurs, the department/divisional leadership and/or DIO/dean need to step in and relieve you of all clinical responsibilities for whatever length of time is needed, without questions. A day or two is woefully inadequate; a week or more is likely needed. As described below, you will need to attend to the grief of a significant number of people (including yourself), and that will require your full presence. Trying to care for patients during such a time is unlikely to be in the patients' best interest. It also sends a message to the residents that taking time to heal is not really important.

Attend to the emotions of your residents
Attending to the emotions of your residents is a bullet point in many of this book's chapters. When a resident in your program dies, you will be called to bear witness to the other residents' grief, depression, guilt, shame, anger, anxiety, trauma, and possibly their own suicidal ideation (McMenamy et al., 2008). Some of these emotions will be hidden emotions, making them harder to address. Being aware of the possible emotions could help you feel more prepared; call on your courage, resilience, and love to get you through.

There will be formal, large group meetings that you will have to run, including the meeting in which you share the news of the resident's death. The AFSP toolkit has helpful resources, including sample scripts for this and other conversations that you will need to have (Dyrbye et al., 2017). Key things to cover in this meeting include basic facts that are known and allowed to be shared (according to the family's wishes), your own feelings, acknowledgment of the residents' feelings, what to expect over the coming days, and strong encouragement to use existing resources such as formal mental health counseling, personal support systems, each other, trusted faculty, peer support programs (McAllister & Trent, 2018) and others. Another PD who experienced the loss of a resident also strongly urges us to be explicit about the difficulties some residents will face in the coming weeks to months as they wrestle with the death of their colleague (Dickey & Cannon, 2018).

As described in "Room for Improvement" earlier in this chapter, there may be other residents who are really struggling because of the death, and you should employ your leadership team (especially chief residents) to proactively look for them. You may already have residents in mind who you are worried about because they had previously known mental health concerns or because they were very close to the resident that died. Be especially aware of behavior changes in individual residents as a sign that they may be struggling (as described in Chapter 3). One-on-one meetings to check in with these residents are a good idea (Dyrbye et al., 2017.).

Grief resulting from deaths such as suicide can be complicated (Gillies & Neimeyer, 2006) and prolonged (Lichtenthal et al., 2004). Survivors who are able to make sense of such a loss may avoid complicated grief symptoms (Currier et al., 2006), which lends support to the recommendation of providing ongoing opportunities for residents to talk about their lost colleague (Dickey & Cannon, 2018).

Attend to the emotions of the leadership group
The chief residents, APDs, and program staff will need the support of yourself and each other. Set aside time to debrief and grieve together. Encourage them to take advantage of mental health and/or peer support resources. Make space in regularly scheduled meetings to check in with your team, at first to grieve and later (in the post-crisis phase) to understand what you can learn from the crisis to make you a stronger team and program. In some programs, one APD is "assigned" a cohort of residents for semi-annual meetings and other mentoring. If one of the APDs was especially close to the resident who died, you may want to reach out separately to them. Finally, remember that seeing your emotions will be important for your team. If it is difficult for you to show your emotions, at least articulate them.

Attend to your own emotions
You need to take time to process your own grief and other emotions (See Chapter 10). All the resources that you recommended for others . . . you need them, too. Do not let the "busyness" of the many crisis-related tasks allow you to push your own feelings aside. And let's be very clear: this was not your fault. Full stop.

Also, realize that you do not have control over the entirety of the message about this resident's death. In the world of online obituaries and social media, you will not be able to control what others say or post, so find your peace in that knowledge.

Attend to the family's grief
The AFSP toolkit describes considerations for talking with the family after a resident has died. One important consideration is whether the family will allow you to disclose the cause of death to the rest of the residents. This conversation is very difficult and will happen over multiple calls or meetings in the days/weeks following the event. In the immediate aftermath, the family may not be ready to share that the resident died by suicide, but keep talking to them. In Annette's case, I had many conversations with her family over the weeks after her death, both by phone and in person. Listening with empathy and patiently continuing the dialogue allowed me to build a genuine, caring relationship with the family. Those efforts eventually led them to see why sharing the truth with the residents was the right course of action. Because Annette's family wanted to prevent this from happening to someone else, they supported our sharing it with the residents and even incorporating the story into our orientation for future interns. Patience, empathy, and caring were the keys. If the family indicates that they blame you, the program, or the institution, you should seek legal advice through the GME office or the institution's risk management group.

Start a dialogue about resident death and suicide with other PDs at your institution
Sharing experiences of resident suicide with other program directors is not common practice. After Annette's death, I discovered that another suicide had occurred in a different GME program at our institution. As a PD community within an institution, I believe that sharing these experiences could help other PDs (in the pre-crisis stage) reflect on their programs and prepare. Additionally, it is incredibly lonely to be the PD in these crises. The other PDs at our institutions are almost like cousins we don't see all that often, but we have a shared background and culture, like an extended family, that makes it instantly easy to relate to each other in hardship. We are missing a rich source of support by not talking with them in these moments. We should design a mechanism to share these moments for the benefit of the PD going through the crisis, as well as for those who are not (yet) going through a crisis. Start by working through the DIO or GME dean and the Graduate Medical Education Committee.

Reassess your program's well-being resources
In the post-crisis phase, you and your leadership team should take account of what resources exist and what you will need to prevent or better cope with future tragedy. When there is a

trainee suicide, everyone focuses on mental health resources (which is important, clearly), but there are often non-mental health stressors (e.g., other health issues, financial concerns, relationship strain) that contribute. All health and wellness issues should be evaluated as possible foci. Designing well-being programming is not always straightforward. My residents often say they want more time off instead of activities that the program plans. However, activities that the program plans are meant to get residents who might be isolated out with their colleagues (which I explain to them every time this comes up). Regardless, having a budget for well-being activities is a good place to start, and now is the time to ask for it. Starting a resident-led wellness committee is another potential intervention.

Talk with your team about programmatic changes you should consider in response to the resident death. For example, should you screen for mental health issues in the residents regularly (e.g., before each semi-annual review)? Are there proactive mental health interventions or reflection exercises that you should consider during curricular time such as group debriefs? For a further discussion of such ideas, see Chapter 5. We know of one program that has each resident invite a significant other/important person to a gathering during intern orientation to talk about the challenges of residency, including the potential for addiction and other mental health concerns. The purpose is to engage someone close to the resident in monitoring well-being and offering support.

Debrief your team processes so that you grow stronger
In the post-crisis phase, use meeting time to debrief the communication and processes your team used during the crisis (see Chapter 1). If a policy existed already, how closely did you follow it? Should adjustments to the policy or composition of the crisis team be made? What did you do well as a team? What could you do better? Not all aspects of this crisis will apply to the next one, but some might. Use this as an opportunity to grow stronger as a team.

Develop a policy for how safety checks are done
This is a step for the post-crisis stage: Consider having a program (or even an institutional) policy about when and how "safety checks" are performed when a resident does not come to work as expected. The practice of sending chief residents to check on absent residents should be relegated to the past. If your GME office does not have a policy and does not wish to pursue one, talk with your campus police. If they do not have the jurisdiction to do such safety checks at the homes of residents, they could connect you to the local police for input. Either

way, having trained professionals do these visits may result in less overall trauma to members of the program than asking chief residents or faculty.

Even without your requesting it, a resident could happen upon a suicide scene because they took it upon themselves to check on a colleague or because of a fluke. Whoever discovers a suicide or other traumatic scene will be significantly affected. They may be plagued by survivor's guilt or guilt that they should have done more or arrived sooner. There is a very real chance that they will contend with PTSD. Be liberal about time off for recovery for these people and connect them right away to available mental health resources.

Work across departments to strengthen resident connections
Having resident connections across programs can build individual networks with positive ripple effects. We have seen this through a GME program that gives small grants for wellness that require at least two programs to participate together (Farkas AH et al., 2023). A great example was a brewery tour/dinner that brought together general surgery and anesthesia residents to get to know each other as people rather than masked (almost de-identified) workers in the OR. We have also seen interprogram tennis tournaments, Wiffle ball games, boat rides, and community volunteer events. With which other programs do your residents frequently interact? Could you and their PD plan an event to bring them together?

Summary

The death of a resident, whether unexpected or due to a prolonged illness, is a terrible tragedy. PDs will have their own emotions even as they play a central role in helping others heal. These tragedies result in sadness, guilt, and sometimes isolation. Working with your leadership team and sharing your feelings with them will help everyone move through their grief. Building a stronger leadership team, making the program stronger, and working across departments or at the institutional level to bring needed change can give PDs purpose in the months after losing a resident.

Table 3. Summary approach to the unexpected death of a resident	
Pre-Crisis	Check with your GME office to determine if a crisis plan exists in case a resident dies unexpectedly
Crisis	Activate a crisis response team
	Assign roles, including your own
	Pause and consider the privacy issues
	Use the mental health resources available
	Clear your calendar
	Attend to the emotions of the residents, leadership team, family, and yourself
Post-Crisis	Plan a memorial
	Consider a broader discussion among other GME leaders at your institution about how other PDs have managed resident deaths
	Assess and ask for resources needed for future prevention/management
	Debrief the crisis response with your team and make adjustments for the future

Citations

Currier, J. M., Holland, J. M., & Neimeyer, R. A. (2006). Sense-Making, Grief, and the Experience of Violent Loss: Toward a Mediational Model. *Death Stud, 30*(5), 403-428. https://doi.org/10.1080/07481180600614351

Dickey, C. C., & Cannon, B. (2018). When a Resident or Fellow Dies. *J Grad Med Educ, 10*(4), 387-391. https://doi.org/10.4300/jgme-d-17-00566.1

Dyrbye, L., Konopasek, L., & Moutier, C. V., for the American Foundation for Suicide Prevention (2017). *After a Suicide: A Toolkit for Physician Residency/Fellowship Programs.* American Foundation for Suicide Prevention. https://www.acgme.org/globalassets/pdfs/13287_afsp_after_suicide_clinician_toolkit_final_2.pdf

Farkas AH, Fletcher KE, Pilarski A, & Syam D. (2023). Well-Being Mini-Awards: Promoting Interdepartmental Connections among Trainees (Abstract). Society of General Internal Medicine National Meeting, Aurora, CO, May 2023.

Gillies, J., & Neimeyer, R. A. (2006). Loss, Grief, and the Search for Significance: Toward a Model of Meaning Reconstruction in Bereavement. *Journal of Constructivist Psychology, 19*(1), 31-65. https://doi.org/10.1080/10720530500311182

Khan, A. (2017). A Death in the Family. *JAMA 318*(16), 1543-1544. https://doi.org/10.1001/jama.2017.13531

Lichtenthal, W. G., Cruess, D. G., & Prigerson, H. G. (2004). A Case for Establishing Complicated Grief as a Distinct Mental Disorder in DSM-V. *Clin Psychol Rev, 24*(6), 637-662. https://doi.org/10.1016/j.cpr.2004.07.002

McAllister, R. K., & Trent, M. (2018). Caring for the Survivors When a Resident or Fellow Dies. *J Grad Med Educ, 10*(6), 719. https://doi.org/10.4300/jgme-d-18-00753.1 McMenamy, J. M., Jordan, J. R., & Mitchell, A. M. (2008). What do Suicide Survivors Tell Us They Need? Results of a Pilot Study. *Suicide Life Threat Behav, 38*(4), 375-389. https://doi.org/10.1521/suli.2008.38.4.375

Yaghmour, N. A., Brigham, T. P., Richter, T., Miller, R. S., Philibert, I., Baldwin, D. C., Jr., & Nasca, T. J. (2017). Causes of Death of Residents in ACGME-Accredited Programs 2000 Through 2014: Implications for the Learning Environment. *Acad Med, 92*(7), 976-983. https://doi.org/10.1097/acm.0000000000001736

CHAPTER 5

Leading through a Crisis on Campus

Matthew Goldblatt, MD

Kathlyn E. Fletcher, MD, MA

Medical College of Wisconsin

Dr. Goldblatt and Dr. Fletcher describe two campus crises that did not directly involve their programs but affected their residents. They learned that adjacent crises need to be actively managed, and that they represent opportunities to support the residents and bring resources that may prevent future crises.

Introduction

Residency programs are interconnected within the academic environment. Some programs are part of vast medical centers with residents, fellows, students, and several hospitals on the same campus while others have fewer or different interconnections. Interconnections often operate in the background, especially when all systems are working well. Interconnections become visible when something is not working or when a crisis occurs. In this chapter, we highlight the ways in which a crisis outside of your program can impact your residents. The cases in this chapter remind us to ask ourselves if an event that seems outside our realm might be affecting our residents.

Story #1: Violent Crime in the Work Environment

We have changed the names of those involved in this story, but we did not change the details because they were reported in the local news.

It was a bitterly cold January morning, and I woke up to a text alert from the medical center that there had been an event requiring a police presence on campus a few hours before. I scanned the news to try to find more details. There were already breaking news stories that reported a death in a parking garage at one of our hospitals. It would be many more hours before the full scope of the tragedy became apparent, and we learned about the details in the same timeframe as the general public. An inpatient advanced practice provider (APP) named Jeannie (not her real name) was leaving the hospital after her evening shift. She walked alone to her car, a usual practice for many people, in a well-lit parking garage attached to the hospital. She approached her car and was struck in the back of the head. The assailant then put her in his car and drove to another area of the parking structure and left her to die in the bitter cold. Jeannie was found sometime later. She was taken to the campus trauma center but was unable to be revived. Within the next 24 hours, word spread around the hospital by both unofficial and official communication that Jeannie was murdered.

Because the details of the events were unknown outside the hospital leadership, rumors started to spread. Was this a random event? Was everyone unsafe? Was the assailant a patient? Employee? The residents, like many other workers at the hospital, were afraid for their safety. Across the hospital, people were also devastated by the loss of a co-worker, especially through an act of violence.

The following day, hospital administration was proactive, sharing as much information as possible while still protecting the rights of the victim and her family. Details of the crime were not made public. However, the local news was reporting her death as a murder.

Advice from the Literature and Practical Wisdom
Recognize that a crisis is occurring

This crisis had a fast onset, but it wasn't clear to me that it was going to be a crisis that affected my program. Because Jeannie was not in our (MG's) department, I did not realize the connection the residents felt with her until they specifically told me. The residents saw themselves as vulnerable because of the parallels between their lives and hers. They were similar ages, worked at similar times of day and at the same place. Therefore, potential for psychological response to Jeannie's story, even without a personal connection, made this a crisis for our program.

Be ready to manage the immediate emotions

Plan time for the residents to be together. The department chair and I organized a departmental meeting for this purpose that included faculty, residents, and hospital administration. Many of my residents had seen Jeannie around the hospital, and many recollected communicating with her about shared patients. The residents expressed an immediate emotional loss, which they discussed at the debriefing.

Recognize different approaches to grieving and provide a range of resources

Some residents respond to trauma by getting back to work and not thinking about it. Others are so preoccupied by their thoughts of the tragedy that they can't work, and there are many between these extremes. Most residents feel that they are stronger than the average person and don't seek help until it is too late, so take this opportunity to remind the residents of resources they can access to promote their own recovery. Such resources may include access to psychologists/psychiatrists. Make it clear that residents can take time away from work if needed. Try to reduce barriers to seeking help such as time, perceived helpfulness, and stigma (Ey et al., 2013). Identifying as male and underrepresented in medicine are associated with decreased likeliness of using resources such as counseling services (Ey et al., 2013).

Residents themselves may be the most important untapped resource in these moments of crisis and grief. We encourage our residents and co-workers to look out for one another and identify others who may be showing signs of stress. Members of a residency family are often very close, and they share a lot of information and insight about each other. They may be the first to become aware of a subtle change in a colleague. Therefore, it is important to make the residents aware of signs of depression and difficulty coping in their colleagues. A group at New York University developed an observed structural evaluation (OSCE) to give interns the opportunity to practice identifying a struggling colleague; they found that many were not prepared (Zabar et al., 2019). Giving residents the tools to talk with each other when they are worried ("embrace the awkward") could be extremely valuable (see Box).

How to start a conversation with someone you are worried about
Advice from David Cipriano, PhD, Director of Student and Resident Behavioral Services, Medical College of Wisconsin 1. Begin by sharing your observations of the person and then take a guess at what underlying feeling is being represented. For example, "You don't seem quite like yourself lately. I'm wondering if you're feeling a little down" or "You've been a little short lately, that's not like you. You seem tense." 2. Follow up with a validating statement and what you are going to do. That might sound like this: "It's no wonder, you've had a lot going on. I'm here for you if you want to talk." Or perhaps this: "Our mood can become depressed after a loss. There's help for this, I'll support you." 3. Consider using some self-disclosure to help the person get past stigma and stoicism. Without making it all about you, give a brief example of a time you struggled in a similar situation. This can be especially powerful when coming from a valued colleague or an esteemed mentor. 4. Once they start talking, keep it going by using reflective statements such as "So, that makes you feel ____" or "I hear how frustrated you are." These statements invite clarification (if you focused on the wrong feeling) and also elaboration on how they are actually feeling. Reflective statements validate the person's feelings as well, which can go a long way toward making the person feel comfortable. 5. You can close the conversation with a reminder of mental health resources that are available at your institution or encouragement to talk with a trusted faculty member about how they are feeling.

Remember that medical and mental health history should not be evaluated/treated by peers or PDs. The role of the PD is to ensure that all the resources are made available and that there is no stigma associated with utilizing them.

Bring the right people to the table to address the residents' concerns

Who will the residents want to hear from after a tragedy? Besides the program leadership, they will likely want to hear from people who can effect change to prevent another event. Our residents were afraid for their safety, and security is typically the job of the hospital. Hospital employees are at the mercy of hospital policy, so having the hospital administration in front of the residents is a powerful tool to show the residents that their concerns are important. Hospital administration listened to the residents' concerns and answered questions honestly.

Several of our services include home call, during which residents may walk into the hospital alone at night. After day shifts, residents sometimes leave the hospital later than intended, when there is no foot traffic on the way to their cars. Residents asked how hospital security would increase patrols and if the residents could call security to have an escort to their cars during off hours. The hospital administration described immediate changes to be made. When they didn't know the answers to questions, they promised to get back to us, and they did.

In our case, the hospital administration quickly increased security patrols and camera surveillance and encouraged using security escorts to cars. The hospital also reassigned parking so that residents who worked at night could park nearest the walkway entrance to the hospital. If your institution is not as quick to provide these resources, this is the time to ask for them. Consider working with other programs and engaging your departmental leadership to provide additional advocacy. In our experience, having departmental chairs at the table helped to convey the seriousness of the concern to hospital administration.

Implement or advocate for short-term changes that are within your control
Your residents will want an immediate plan to ensure their safety, and some interventions are not within your direct power. If not already available, advocate for security escorts to cars at night. If already available, alert your residents to that resource. Many hospitals have escort policies, but these documents (or electronic files) may be difficult to locate. As a PD, you can find and distribute these policies. If these resources do not exist or are not together in a place easily accessed by the residents, work with the hospital or the GME office to collate and widely share them.

Some college campuses offer a virtual escort app for their students who walk alone at night. They use GPS to determine the student's location and if they start to run. In addition, sensors within the phone can signal events that could represent an attack, such as headphones being pulled out, the phone dropping, or the person falling. At the time of this writing, these apps can be found by searching for "virtual escort app." Some results include the following: Rave Guardian, Pathlight, and LiveSafe. None of these apps have been evaluated by the authors. Potential downsides include draining the phone's battery and the possible sharing of private information.

Other needed changes cannot be made immediately, but you can still advocate for them.

Hospitals can hire more security personnel, add security cameras and emergency alert stations, increase security patrols, and build barriers like automatic gates.

Finally, re-evaluate the security practices at other sites where your residents rotate. Communicate with their security offices about the incident so that they are prepared for an increase in requests for escorts. Circle back to the residents to reassure them that you are considering the big picture and preventing future problems.

Ask for more resources
In the post-crisis phase of a situation like this one, take the time to assess what resources could have potentially prevented the event from occurring or would have helped you manage the aftermath better; then leverage your experience to amass what you need.

If your program has only bare-bones mental health resources, this is an ideal opportunity to ask for expanded services to implement in the post-crisis phase and carry over to the pre-crisis phase. Easy access to affordable mental health services is required by the ACGME and explained in the Learning and Working Environment section of the Common Program Requirements (Accreditation Council for Graduate Medical Education, 2022). Some residencies have implemented "opt-out" mental health appointments for residents as a way to reduce the stigma attached to accessing care (Sofka et al., 2018). Residents who have attended initial opt-out sessions report more willingness to seek help through the employee assistance program in the future (Sofka et al., 2018). In another study, 25% of interns who attended an opt-out mental health session subsequently sought care (Major et al., 2021). Therefore, residents may be more likely to access mental health services in an actual crisis if they have attended opt-out sessions beforehand (Batra et al., 2018).

Peer support programs are another preventative option for the pre-crisis period (Abrams, 2017). One program at our institution implemented monthly discussion groups facilitated by a faculty psychiatrist, which may require departmental resources. The goal was to provide time and space for healthy debriefing about the stress of residency. These programs can increase self-compassion, hope, and belongingness (Jain et al., 2022). Senior residents or alumni participation may be helpful (Jain et al., 2022). If a formal peer support program is not feasible, consider training your senior residents to debrief acute stressors such as patient deaths. Interns find it helpful when senior residents debrief difficult situations, especially when residents talk about their own emotional reactions (Moore et al., 2020).

Take care of your team

In the post-crisis phase, check on the emotional status of your leadership team. While you and your leadership team have been attending to the needs of your resident constituents, your team members may not have been attending to their own fear, anger, and grief. If you have regular leadership meetings, dedicate one to debriefing the event and supporting each other. If you think anyone needs additional help, consider reaching out to them separately to encourage them to seek the help they need.

Story #2: On-campus suicide of a resident from a different program

We have changed the names of those involved in this story, but we did not change the details because they were reported in the local news.

An uneventful holiday weekend was drawing to a close when I received a text page from one of my chief residents. Part of the hospital was on lockdown, and it was not clear why. The locked-down area included several resident call rooms and some of the operating room suites. At the time, the residents did not have their own lounges or common areas, so most of the residents who were sheltering in place were alone. There was a rumor that someone was armed in that part of the hospital. It was a harrowing few hours as little information was available, even to those who were sheltering in place. Eventually, the story began to trickle out.

Darrin, a resident from a different program at our institution, had died by suicide in the hospital. Clinical activities in that area were shut down pending an investigation. The news and rumors spread quickly.

As the days and weeks progressed, it became apparent that mental illness, life stress, workplace stress, and access to potentially lethal means created the perfect storm. Many co-workers had recognized that Darrin had been having problems. As often is the case in these situations, no one thought that he would take his life.

In the weeks to months after this event, the hospital created resident-specific common areas for respite, quiet time, and nourishment throughout the hospital. Outreach between mental health and residency programs increased and continued beyond this event.

Advice from the Literature and Practical Wisdom

Suicide is the second-leading cause of death in residents, second only to malignancy, and followed by accidents (some of which may also be suicides) (Yaghmour et al., 2017). Residents and faculty have a deep knowledge of many potent drugs. By virtue of their work, residents from particular programs also have access to drugs that if self-administered could be lethal. Nights and weekends in the hospital often represent significantly decreased staffing levels and oversight. This case represents the perfect storm: night, weekend, stress, mental health issues, access to lethal means. How to lead through a suicide in your own program is covered in Chapter 4.

Be ready to have an immediate response
Within 24 hours (or sooner), reach out to your residents and brief them on the facts as they are known. These moments are difficult because there may not be an official report from the institution, and the institution may even tell leaders not to discuss the event with their constituents. There are privacy concerns for the family of the resident who died, and no one in program leadership wants to spread rumors. However, in our experience, saying nothing makes the residents in your program furious, anxious, and distrustful. We advise having an in-person meeting to avoid the establishment of a written record of the event, which may ultimately be proven wrong. Another advantage to an in-person meeting is the opportunity to judge how your residents are coping.

The residents want you to tell them everything, which is usually not possible. The second-best option is to share the best information that you have available. If you have information that you are not allowed to share for legal or other reasons, be honest that you are not able to share everything at present but that you realize how frustrating that is (see Room for Improvement).

Provide emotional support
Be prepared to provide your residents with all available support (see Story #1 above). Most residents have likely heard that mental health care is available to them, but they may not know how to access it. Reduce stigma by encouraging residents to access mental health care. Make it easy by giving out laminated index cards listing phone numbers and resources so that residents can put them in their white coat pockets or hang them on their work lockers. Consider including a footnote in routine emails listing crisis line numbers.

As in the previous scenario, it is important for colleagues and co-workers to keep an eye out for one another. You do not want to create a scenario where co-workers are reporting on one another, but the buddy system can help a person in crisis know that someone is looking out for them. Often in cases like this, when people who know the victim look back, there were subtle signs of a problem. Give residents the tools to talk to co-workers when they are concerned about them.

Here is a great example of residents looking out for each other. A few months after the suicide, a PD colleague was contacted by one of her senior residents who was concerned for the safety of a resident from another program rotating on their team. The senior resident described a written note he had found that referenced despair and dying. The PD expressed appreciation for the resident's caring and courage in contacting her, and they discussed a strategy. The PD called the other resident's PD right away to relay the concerns and offered to talk about options together.

Identify and advocate for missing resources

Ask for resources aimed at preventing future tragedies. When tragedies occur adjacent to your program, the resources to ask/advocate for might be hospital-wide rather than specific to your program. Are there opportunities for the hospital to do something for all trainees? For example, most hospitals have call rooms for the residents but do not have touchdown spaces where they can go and step away from the constant pressures of taking care of sick patients, the never-ending pages, and other care team members stopping by to discuss issues. Private respite spaces where residents can be with other residents to decompress are important. If such space does not exist at your site, work with other PDs or your GME office to advocate for it. It will take time to create, but planning can be initiated immediately, which will positively impact the residents.

In our case, the hospital prioritized plans for three large resident spaces to be shared among residency programs. The plans included touchdown work areas and gathering spaces with kitchenettes. Individual residency programs also designed smaller spaces for the sole use of their residents. These spaces came to fruition over three years and have been a great contributor to resident wellness.

On a smaller scale, in the wake of the resident suicide, one department chair reversed a previous decision about supporting occasional resident lunches. He re-engaged in talks with the PD to plan six lunches a year that were only focused on being together. He cited as a reason realizing that residents might benefit from more casual touchpoints with their peers and program leadership.

Room for Improvement

Because the suicide described in Story #2 occurred on a holiday weekend, I (KF) was out of town. Additionally, the GME office had sent an email to PDs telling us not to say anything to our residents until we had official word about what had happened. So, I did not reach out to the residents at all. They were confused and angry. Some of them had sheltered in place during the night of the suicide. All of them needed to debrief. That was a real miss.

In retrospect, I should have trusted my leadership team to manage the situation in my absence. An APD on campus could have led an in-person meeting with the residents. The APD could have shared that we did not have any official information, but we wanted them to have time to express their grief over losing a peer and the chance to debrief about the shelter-in-place order.

Summary

When a crisis occurs close to your program, there may not be an obvious connection between the crisis and your residents. It is best to assume that there is a connection so that you do not delay recovery. You need to be in front of the residents with information, reassurance, and emotional support. If there is a potential threat to the residents' safety, address it honestly and bring in the leaders who have the power to make necessary changes. Use these opportunities to prepare your residents for future crises, especially from a mental health perspective. Finally, assess your program's resources and ask for what you may need to prevent or respond to a similar crisis.

Table 1. Summary approach to campus crises	
Pre-Crisis	Recognize the onset of the crisis and communicate it to the residents
Crisis	Communicate what you can even if it isn't as much as the residents want Take care of the residents' immediate emotions
Post-Crisis	Engage leaders with the power to effect change Assure the safety of the residents Assess the needs of the residents and deploy resources to support them Ask for missing resources

Citations

Abrams, M. P. (2017). Improving Resident Well-Being and Burnout: The Role of Peer Support. *J Grad Med Educ*, 9(2), 264. https://doi.org/10.4300/jgme-d-16-00805.1

Accreditation Council for Graduate Medical Education. (2022). *ACGME - Common Program Requirements (Residency)*. https://www.acgme.org/globalassets/PFAssets/ProgramRequirements/CPRResidency_2022v2.pdf

Batra, M., McPhillips, H., & Shugerman, R. (2018). Improving Resident Use of Mental Health Resources: It's Time for an Opt-Out Strategy to Address Physician Burnout and Depression (Commentary). J Grad Med Educ, 10(1), 67-69. https://doi.org/10.4300/jgme-d-17-00941.1

Ey, S., Moffit, M., Kinzie, J. M., Choi, D., & Girard, D. E. (2013). "If You Build It, They Will Come": Attitudes of Medical Residents and Fellows about Seeking Services in a Resident Wellness Program. *J Grad Med Educ*, 5(3), 486-492. https://doi.org/10.4300/jgme-d-12-00048.1

Jain, A., Tabatabai, R., Schreiber, J., Vo, A., & Riddell, J. (2022). "Everybody in this Room Can Understand": A Qualitative Exploration of Peer Support during Residency Training. *AEM Educ Train*, 6(2), e10728. https://doi.org/10.1002/aet2.10728

Major, A., Williams, J. G., McGuire, W. C., Floyd, E., & Chacko, K. (2021). Removing Barriers: A Confidential Opt-Out Mental Health Pilot Program for Internal Medicine Interns. *Acad Med*, 96(5), 686-689. https://doi.org/10.1097/acm.0000000000003965

Moore, K. A., O'Brien, B. C., & Thomas, L. R. (2020). "I Wish They Had Asked": A Qualitative Study of Emotional Distress and Peer Support During Internship. *J Gen Intern Med*, 35(12), 3443-3448. https://doi.org/10.1007/s11606-020-05803-4

Sofka, S., Grey, C., Lerfald, N., Davisson, L., & Howsare, J. (2018). Implementing a Universal Well-Being Assessment to Mitigate Barriers to Resident Utilization of Mental Health Resources. *J Grad Med Educ*, 10(1), 63-66. https://doi.org/10.4300/jgme-d-17-00405.1

Yaghmour, N. A., Brigham, T. P., Richter, T., Miller, R. S., Philibert, I., Baldwin, D. C., Jr., & Nasca, T. J. (2017). Causes of Death of Residents in ACGME-Accredited Programs 2000 Through 2014: Implications for the Learning Environment. *Acad Med*, 92(7), 976-983. https://doi.org/10.1097/acm.0000000000001736

Zabar, S., Hanley, K., Horlick, M., Cocks, P., Altshuler, L., Watsula-Morley, A., Berman, R., Hochberg, M., Phillips, D., Kalet, A., & Gillespie, C. (2019). "I Cannot Take This Any More!": Preparing Interns to Identify and Help a Struggling Colleague. *Journal of General Internal Medicine*, 34(5), 773-777. https://doi.org/10.1007/s11606-019-04886-y

CHAPTER 6

Leading Through Community Tragedy

Mark Rasnake, MD
University of Central Florida College of Medicine

Glenn Paetow, MD, MACM
Hennepin County Medical Center

Kathlyn E. Fletcher, MD, MA
Medical College of Wisconsin

In this chapter, the authors explore two very different community tragedies: a hurricane and a violent death that resulted in national protests. Both require attention to the involvement of individual residents, the program, and the community. Both require courage, empathy, patience, and grace to navigate these situations.

Introduction

Tragedies in our local communities are far too common. From natural disasters to mass shootings, our communities absorb a variety of terrible events. The effect of community tragedies on graduate medical education programs is related to both professional and personal factors, such as who the victims were, whether our residents were involved in the care of patients affected, and whether any residents were directly affected.

Story #1: Hurricane Ian

September 22, 2022: The fall meeting for the Association of Program Directors in Internal Medicine was in San Diego, and I was there, knowing a storm was brewing close to home in the Gulf of Mexico. The storm was steering well away from Naples, where my program is located, and was forecast to hit much further north, past Tampa Bay. By the time the conference ended and my red-eye flight arrived home early-morning September 25, the storm track had shifted sharply toward Naples. Our hospital, a half mile from the ocean, now was facing potential storm impact. We had to prepare hastily.

My program is a community-based program of 48 residents. We had just graduated our third class of residents when Hurricane Ian began its path toward us. During the last storm to impact our area (Hurricane Irma in 2017), the program was new; the first class of 16 interns was only in its third month of training. The default response of the hospital during Irma was to send the interns home and cover the hospital with faculty until the "all clear." As Ian approached, not involving the residents was still the plan, even though we now had a mature program with seasoned senior residents. We hastily revised our plans to have in-house and standby teams of residents help cover our share of the patient load. Our leadership group decided that I would stay home on the day of the storm, and one chief resident plus eight PGY2/PGY3 residents would stay at the hospital with the supervising hospital medicine faculty.

When I awoke the next day (Tuesday) at 5:00 AM, the Weather Channel radar showed the storm just southwest of us. I had been living in Florida for less than a year, and this was my family's first storm. The uncertainty was stressful, despite having everything on the hurricane readiness list.

It was a substantial, slow-moving storm. I spoke to the chief resident at the hospital just before high tide, so I knew the hospital wasn't flooding at that point. Shortly thereafter, we lost power (around 11:00 AM), and I lost communication with the hospital. I felt unsettled at home while my residents were at the hospital, but hospital leadership had assured me I wasn't needed on-site. The eye passed due west of us early that afternoon, bringing the worst of the wind and rain to our neighborhood. Ian later made landfall in the nearby Fort Myers area.

Near sunset, the winds died down enough for us to venture outside and assess the damage to our neighborhood. Fortunately, our house was not directly impacted, but we felt the pain and worry for others, and for the community we love, knowing many lives and places would be forever altered.

Travel was extremely difficult for the first few days after the storm due to non-functioning traffic lights, downed trees, and lack of open gas stations. I made it to the hospital on Wednesday morning to check on the residents who had been there overnight. Resident roles had been limited to caring for patients already in-house, as there were no new hospital admissions during the storm.

The residents said they were not worried about their physical safety because they trusted the robustness of the facility and knew that they were not in the direct line of the storm. They were most worried about the community at large and what would happen to our training program. There was no cell service in our area for several days, leading to significant logistical difficulties contacting and coordinating return times with our relief teams. It took about 48 hours before the last of the "storm" residents went home from the hospital.

Fortunately, most residents lived far enough inland that they were spared any direct storm damage. However, several residents lost their apartments, vehicles, and/or belongings, as did several of our core faculty members. Hospital teams helped our staff, including the residents, navigate the Federal Emergency Management Agency (FEMA) assistance programs and insurance issues. Our chiefs also established a GoFundMe page to get quick financial help to residents who had lost belongings. Displaced residents stayed with faculty or other residents ("buddy care" saved the day); no one had to go to shelters.

Our hospital lost external power for three weeks, but we operated inpatient services at 100% with generators. Unfortunately, clinics remained closed until external power was restored. For several weeks after the storm, our hospital's clinical volume was lower, as many retirees and vacationers avoided the area. By December, we had returned to normal.

Advice from the Literature and Practical Wisdom
Announce the onset of the crisis

Communicate the onset of the crisis to your program and leadership group. With a hurricane, state authorities will determine the onset through evacuation notices, etc. You should activate your program's crisis plan in conjunction with the hospital's crisis plan. Our hospital leadership had been through storms before and knew what to expect. They communicated frequently with all hospital staff leading up to the storm. The chief residents and I communicated directly with the residents, taking the hospital messages and distilling the department-specific information for them. Note that some residents will experience pre-storm anxiety, and your messaging should acknowledge and normalize it.

Assemble your emergency team

Once you determine that you will have residents in the hospital during the emergency, put your team together. We recommend starting with a team of volunteers; we had plenty. Ask for more volunteers than you need for one shift, so they can take turns resting, if necessary. We decided to use only PGY2 and PGY3 residents. Depending on your program and the time of year, including interns may be reasonable.

Work with the hospital leadership to ascertain the supervision plan for the residents. If you anticipate that communication with those outside the hospital will be compromised, in-house supervision will be necessary. For us (an internal medicine program), a hospitalist and a chief resident served as attendings. In some specialties, chief residents do not have faculty status. If you are leading a surgical program, who would supervise an emergency surgery?

Assess and amass resources

Consider the space available in the hospital for the emergency teams to work and sleep. This may require coordinating with other departments that plan to have residents and/or faculty there. Do the workspaces/call rooms all have emergency power? If not, where will your team spend time if regular power is lost?

If there is time to let the emergency team go home and collect their personal emergency supplies, they should do so. Backup batteries for cell phones are especially important for communication. Nearly 25% of the state of Florida lost power during Hurricane Ian, so backup batteries are essential (Livingston, 2022). Verify what resources (such as food) the hospital will be able to provide for workers.

Trust your team

Once you have planned for the looming crisis, trust the team you have put in place. Our chief residents are used to responding to minor crises, so I handed the reins to the chief who stayed in the hospital. This is easier if you have established trust in your leadership group and have shared mental models of teamwork and individual responsibility. I stayed in touch with the emergency team as best I could during and after the storm. I got back to the hospital as soon as it was safe, but I trusted them to manage whatever arose in the interim.

Anticipate communication issues during and after the crisis

We rely on the cell phone network as both a primary and backup means of communication. A true backup is necessary for emergencies that threaten cell phone towers or that may overwhelm network capacity (Table 1). In our case, our chief resident used text messaging, which uses less bandwidth than phone calls (Ready.gov, 2023). He also used WhatsApp, social media, and email. Most programs have social media accounts such as Instagram. Its primary use may be recruitment, but an auxiliary use is emergency communication. Residents should follow the program's social media as an emergency communication strategy. If electronic communication isn't possible because of infrastructure issues, residents should report to a specific meeting point when safe travel is possible. This will facilitate in-person communication of assignments and accounting for all team members.

Table 1. Communication strategies during natural disasters
<ul><li>Text</li><li>Social media</li><li>Email (institution-based and personal)</li><li>Internet-based apps such as WhatsApp</li><li>Pre-arranged, in-person meeting time/place (maybe have two, just in case)</li></ul>

Align work with resources and need in the post-crisis phase

Take time to assess your workforce, its needs, and the needs of the community once the danger has passed. You may need to realign your workforce, so be ready to reassign residents based on community need and availability of both residents and rotations (Table 2).

Table 2. Post-natural disaster workforce alignment considerations	
Question	**Considerations**
What is the state of the medical center?	• Structural damage to hospital or clinic buildings that do not allow for patient care
What is the availability of the residents?	• Residents with damage/property loss • Evacuated residents
What are the needs of the residents?	• Housing • Loss of essential belongings • Childcare needs
What are the needs of the community?	• Medical care for injuries (immediate) • Care for illness post-crisis (weeks-months) (e.g. storm water–associated infection after floods; fungal infections after tornadoes)
What rotations need additional support?	• Specific services overwhelmed by patients • Longer-term care patients with nowhere to go for rehabilitation needs • New medical problems arising from the crisis
What rotations will be suspended?	• Operations that are not running • Expected timeline of re-openings (e.g., clinics, wards, operating suites)

Assess your program's needs

The hospital workforce is also affected by community tragedy, including the residents, staff, and faculty. Assess their needs and identify issues that the program can help or influence. Our chief residents started a GoFundMe account for residents who had losses in the storm. They also helped coordinate a "buddy care" system that paired residents who needed housing with residents who could house them. Our outpatient clinics closed temporarily, and we deployed some residents whose outpatient rotations were canceled to help other residents with storm cleanup. Resources from federal and volunteer agencies will likely be available, so communicate their availability to the residents. If hospital resources are available to employees, make sure the residents are eligible for them, too.

Recognize post-storm mental health problems in colleagues and residents

Some people experience post-traumatic stress disorder (PTSD)–like symptoms after hurricanes. As the PD, you do not need to be adept at managing PTSD, but you should be aware that it could happen. Remind your leadership team to be watchful. If you notice that someone is experiencing greater-than-expected anxiety, you can reassure them it is not unusual in the wake of a storm (American Psychological Association, 2011). The APA notes that "abnormal reactions are a normal reaction to an abnormal situation" (American Psychological Association, 2011). Some may need formal counseling, but reassurance and relaxation techniques may suffice for others (American Psychological Association, 2011). If you suspect a true diagnosis of PTSD, psychiatric referral is necessary.

Room for Improvement

Review and update crisis response policies

Reviewing program policies is not a favorite pastime of most PDs, but it must be done. If you are in a region with predictable seasonal crises, review your crisis plans annually before the season. Share updates with your residents and electronically post crisis plans in a drive that your residents can easily find. If your region does not have seasonal crises, set a yearly date to review your general crisis plan.

Create an emergency supply kit for residents who may be stranded in the hospital

We did not have supplies set aside for residents during Hurricane Ian, and our team was in the hospital for two days/nights. Residents should bring their own emergency kit so they have medications and other personal items, including food and water (Ready.gov). Make sure they have their hospital ID. A hospital-based emergency kit (Table 3) could be stored in a chief resident office or other program space until needed.

Table 3. Hospital emergency supply kit for resident teams

- Extra nonperishable foods and water
- Mats for extra sleeping space
- Extra scrubs
- Battery-powered radio
- Extra batteries
- Soap, hand sanitizer, moist towelettes, disinfectant wipes
- Backup cell phone batteries
- Extra blankets, linens, towels
- Toothbrushes and toothpaste
- Pens and paper
- Entertainment items (puzzles, colored pencils, board games)

Encourage the residents to prepare for a disaster

Since Ian, we dedicate curricular time in July for disaster medicine (Table 4). We encourage our residents to develop an individual crisis management plan that includes their family and pets. We also highlight our professional role during crises, including the option to obtain additional training to be better prepared to help. CDC TRAIN is an excellent resource for a variety of courses (Public Health Foundation, 2024). Depending on your location, you could tailor your messaging to hurricanes, tornadoes, earthquakes, etc. Many of our interns are new to hurricane-prone areas and need guidance; start at Ready.gov.

Table 4. Outline of disaster medicine talk
1. Definitions of disaster and disaster medicine
2. Personal preparedness • Preparing yourself and your family
3. Professional preparedness • Consider additional training opportunities to be able to assist in disasters common to your region • Be ready to join a surge team in a disaster
4. What to expect after natural disasters
5. What to expect after man-made disasters (wars, terrorism, transportation, industrial)
6. How to triage/treat patients with acute injuries (chemical, biologic, radiologic, nuclear, explosive, and post-disaster infectious diseases)

Develop your post-storm plan in advance

We did not have a strong post-storm plan for the residency after Ian, but we do now. The first step is the meeting place. Make sure everyone knows where and when to meet after the storm has passed. Identify two meeting locations in case one is not accessible. Second, institute a phone tree to relay messages and to account for everyone.

Instructions to phone tree users
In the event of a recall, the PD or program coordinator will notify the chief residents to begin the recall chain. Contact the person below you, pass along the message, and note who has been contacted before you and who was not reachable. Do not break the chain. If the person below you does not respond, continue down the list until you contact someone. The person at the bottom of the chain then contacts the chief resident at the top of their chain, noting who has been contacted and who is unaccounted for. The chief residents will then pass this information to the PD or coordinator.

Summary

Residents may be both healthcare workers and victims in natural and human-made disasters. Your leadership group should be aware of both and quickly identify needs of the residents and the community. Establish alternative mechanisms for communication, including a planned meeting place/time after the expected end of the disaster so that residents can be accounted for and assigned roles. Resilience, caring, and organization are the essential character traits of the PD in such moments.

Table 5. Summary approach to community disasters	
Pre-Crisis	<ul><li>Review and update relevant program policies</li><li>Remind residents to create emergency kits</li><li>Consider creating a program emergency kit</li><li>Recognize the onset of the crisis and communicate it to the residents</li><li>Establish crisis team (if indicated)</li></ul>
Crisis	<ul><li>Enact the crisis plan</li><li>Remind the residents of the phone tree/recall roster</li><li>Communicate the post-crisis meeting place to the leadership team and residents</li><li>Engage campus support, including the GME office</li></ul>
Post-Crisis	<ul><li>Determine the safety and whereabouts of the residents</li><li>Assess the needs of the residents and deploy resources to support them</li><li>Prepare to redeploy residents to help with community need and to align with available medical center services</li><li>Be aware of post-crisis, PTSD-like syndromes</li></ul>

Story #2: When Community Tragedy Enters Your Emergency Department

One night everything was normal, and the next night it wasn't.

May 25, 2020, began as a typical day in the Hennepin County Medical Center Emergency Department. An ambulance arrived with a 46-year-old African American man in cardiac arrest, accompanied by police. Having police in our ED was not unusual. The ED team tried to resuscitate the patient, but unfortunately, he died. The team moved on to the next patient, but as each hour passed, it became clearer that the patient accompanied by the police was a unique case. Twelve hours later, we had local law enforcement, the Minnesota Bureau of Criminal Apprehension, and hospital administration in the ED, launching an investigation. Quickly, the hospital legal team took over all communication about the case. The patient was George Floyd. It was no longer a typical night.

The immediate aftermath of George Floyd's death impacted our ED programs because the physician who ran the resuscitation was a soon-to-be-graduating senior resident, Brad (name not changed as it was reported in the national news) (Bogel-Burroughs, 2021). Brad quickly became the center of the maelstrom. He spent countless hours over the following weeks in a room with investigators and the hospital legal team. While the hospital DIO was present, the residency program was not a part of those meetings. Closed-door meetings, the ongoing investigation, and patient privacy complicated our ability to offer moral support to our senior resident. It was an enormous amount of personal stress, but he bore it with equanimity. While the residency program offered to free him from clinical duties so he could focus on the legal case, the COVID-19 pandemic was in full swing, and he saw it as his community duty to keep working in the overwhelmed ED. His close-knit social support system rallied around him. He graduated that summer, but the hospital continued to work with him in preparation for what was to come. Between a string of ED shifts at his first job as a newly minted attending, he testified in the Derek Chauvin trial on April 5, 2021, nearly a year after George Floyd's death. The other residents knew that it could have just as easily been one of them in the spotlight. Even after three years, residents sometimes say, "Is this going to end up on the national stage? Will I get subpoenaed for this?" Not every resident would be as well prepared to manage a similar scenario.

In the subsequent months, the unrest in Minneapolis became another source of fear and trauma for the broader Hennepin County Medical Center community. The hospital was boarded up for protection. Armed members of the National Guard were stationed at each corner around the hospital. We could see Minneapolis burning through the ICU windows, and a smoky haze hung over the city. Many employees were afraid of walking to their cars and began using the skywalks and tunnels usually reserved for winter walking. Some chose to sleep at the hospital rather than drive home after the city's curfew. Protesters destroyed businesses, including some close to the hospital. Unexpected highway closures added to the chaos. It felt like a war zone.

In the ED, it was especially difficult. Protesters attacked ambulances, and we feared for the safety of our EMS colleagues as they brought us patients. When patients came to the hospital, security *rushed them in, then closed and guarded the doors immediately to protect the healthcare workers inside. Every time we heard of a police officer shooting, we felt a fresh wave of fear.*

But we didn't just experience fear that summer; we felt moral injury. We viewed ourselves as an anti-racist organization, a place with a history of working on behalf of marginalized communities. We considered ourselves part of the solution. It hurt to realize that many in the community viewed us as part of the system of oppression. The contrast with the very recent "healthcare heroes" era at the beginning of the COVID-19 pandemic made it even more difficult.

With distance, we have come to see the need for intentional community healing. The hospital and the program have renewed their efforts to be part of the healing process. It is an ongoing process, but we are all moving forward.

Advice from the Literature and Practical Wisdom

Take care of the residents who took care of the victim

It is always hard to witness human suffering or death. In a community tragedy, the frontline healthcare team will need support. Check in with residents involved in the care of the victims. As described in previous chapters, know the institutional and program resources available and remind the residents to use them. Make it easy for the residents to take time off to deal with the trauma of being involved.

Consider holding a residency-wide meeting to debrief, as other residents may also have trouble processing the tragedy. Remind your residents to look out for each other (See Chapters 4 and 5 for additional ideas).

Know what happens when a resident gets subpoenaed

If one of your residents receives a subpoena, they will need some just-in-time education (see Reiley et al., 2003, for a good resource). You should also notify your GME office and the hospital risk manager immediately. In our case, the hospital legal team prepared the resident for all legal proceedings, including his eventual court appearance; their involvement was essential. Residents act under the supervision of attending physicians, so it is reasonable to ask if the resident should, or must, be the one to go through depositions and appear in court. If the resident must be part of the process, ensure the active support of the GME office and the hospital legal team.

Recognize your own feelings about the tragedy
You will have your own reaction to community tragedies. Your feelings deserve attention and debriefing, too. You are part of the community in which the tragedy occurred. Take time to name your feelings and know that some days will be dominated by grief, despair, or other emotions. Talk to others, write about your feelings, and seek help if needed. Know that others are having similar feelings. Being open about your feelings may help others recover, too. Chapter 10 has more suggestions about how to care for yourself in such moments.

Recognize the community response to the tragedy
Understand that the community reaction to the tragedy has something to teach the medical community about what matters and how the medical community's role is perceived. In this case, the violence aimed at the ambulances and the hospital emotionally devastated many of us. It took months for us to navigate our own feelings and reach a new understanding of how we would have to change to be part of the solution.

Be part of the community solution
After a tragedy like George Floyd, a mass shooting, or another act of senseless violence, your community needs to heal. The medical center will not be the main player in the healing, but it can influence the healing. Small efforts matter, such as signage declaring an institutional commitment to anti-racism. Large efforts, such as institutional-community partnerships that include investments in the local community, take longer but have deeper impact (Tanzilo, 2023).

Programmatic involvement in the community healing process is possible. Our program already had a robust diversity, equity, and inclusion curriculum. We added additional efforts aimed at integrating the residents with the community. We take our interns on a "mural tour" around Minneapolis to see murals celebrating different cultural groups represented in our city. The tour ends at the George Floyd Memorial. Think about what landmarks your interns could visit that would introduce them to the multicultural aspects of your city. Plan excursions to other culturally diverse parts of the city. We also organize small-group dinners for residents at a Somali restaurant. The residents are usually the only patrons who are not native Somali speakers. They also may be the only non-Somalis in the restaurant (Paetow et al., 2023). One of our interpreters leads the dinner discussion. I realized that the community had noticed this effort when a patient recently asked if we were "the doctors" from the medical center who had dined at the Somali restaurant.

Story #2a: Navigating the Black Lives Matter (BLM) Protests in Milwaukee

In the summer of 2020, the BLM movement rose to international attention as protests grew in number and size. Most protests were peaceful. In some cities, including Milwaukee, curfews were imposed to keep people off the streets at night. In Milwaukee, as in other cities, the local chapter of White Coats for Black Lives organized events, and many of our residents and program leaders participated. I had never participated in a protest before, and I felt the power of coming together with others to express my personal support of the cause. The act of participating in a public protest felt meaningful. I think it mattered to the residents that I and other residency leaders were there.

Advice from the Literature and Practical Wisdom

The BLM protests required nuanced program responses, depending on the local situation. The riots and violence in Minneapolis were very different from the mostly peaceful protests in Milwaukee, and consequently the leadership response at the residency program level was different.

Recognize that a crisis is starting

As a PD, I was caught off guard by how George Floyd's death and the BLM movement turned into a crisis and by the desire of residents to hear from me. In the conceptual framework, we note the importance of recognizing that a crisis is starting. Sometimes the onset is not perfectly clear. One clue to recognizing a crisis is brewing is that you *personally* are feeling uncomfortable about a situation. Notice when you feel grief, fear, discomfort, or uncertainty. Name the emotion, at least in your own mind. If you are feeling that way, others are, too.

Communicate with your residents

Once you realize what you (and likely others) are feeling, say something to your residents. Drafting an email to your program about these moments is HARD, especially because so many situations feel political. Why can't the ACGME require speech writers for program directors? Of course, these emails cannot officially represent your organization. They are still worth writing.

A reasonable approach to this email is to speak for yourself and not on behalf of your team. Depending on the timing and the need to get in front of the situation, you may choose to speak for yourself only. Additionally, if you think that your team is not on the same page (i.e., lacks cohesiveness), then speaking for yourself is a reasonable choice. Our department and program had already begun some work to increase our recruitment of underrepresented residents, so we had spent time in the pre-crisis phase developing cohesiveness applicable to this crisis.

After George Floyd died, it took me days to write something meaningful (see "Room for Improvement" below). When I did address it via email (Box 2), only my program coordinator responded. The radio silence that sometimes comes after these moments of trying to rise to the occasion can be lonely. Still, it is the right thing to do, and it takes courage, humility, and honesty.

Statement about George Floyd emailed to internal medicine residents
I know that many are struggling during this crisis of injustice that is evolving in the country. In your essays about COVID-19, many of you highlighted the inequality and injustice that the pandemic was bringing into the light. Now with another terrible example in the death of George Floyd, I suspect you are feeling this even more acutely. Please look out for one another. Please stand up for one another. Please ask for help if you need it. Remember that [our institution] has mental health resources and the VA is continuing to offer virtual drop-in sessions, too. We have a peer support program with residents trained to help. I thought the emails on Sunday from [institutional] leadership were well thought out, too, and reaffirmed our commitment to dismantling structural racism . . .

Know that there is a very good chance not everyone is on the same page. Assume that some people agree with you, some feel the opposite, many are in between, and some do not care at all.

Take the pulse of your program
It may be helpful to ask your residents how they feel. An approach that I have found helpful is to send an anonymous, open-ended survey question with several days to respond. This gives them time to reflect on how they feel and the space to be honest. We used this approach in July 2020 by sending the residents a few open-ended questions about the impact of the BLM protests on their lives. We used their anonymous reflections as a jumping off point to discuss the issues of social justice and racial inequity inside and outside our program (Patnaik et al., 2022). This exercise showed us the spectrum of feelings in our program, and it galvanized some residents to become more active in anti-racism work (Pallok & Sekhri, 2020).

Keep your residents safe

There are practical considerations to some crises that need to be addressed. When Milwaukee instituted a curfew, the residents needed proof that they were required to be at the hospital to travel there within curfew hours. Hospitals probably know that they need to provide this to their workers, but as a program director, you may need to advocate for residents to receive whatever documentation they need in case law enforcement stops them. I worried about the residents of color in my program and what would happen if they were pulled over by the police during this tenuous time. One of the fellows at our institution had just written an essay that described such an incident from his teenage years (Nunley, 2020).

Room for Improvement

Focus on getting better when you don't get it right

I did not directly address the murder of George Floyd with the residents until eight days after it happened, and I am still not sure why. Being in the racial majority probably played a role in my failure to recognize the importance of the moment. The American Association of Medical Colleges (AAMC) reports that less than 10% of faculty in US medical schools are underrepresented (Association of American Medical Colleges, 2016) and, accordingly, few PDs are underrepresented (Garrison, 2019; O'Connor et al., 2023; Whetstone, 2023; Kalra et al., 2022). George Floyd and the BLM protests may have been especially difficult for non-URM PDs like me to navigate. That left some residents feeling their programs did not realize the importance of the moment. Alec O'Connor, a PD colleague, shared his insight with me:

> *"Sometimes it's obvious, but sometimes some of the residency community perceives something as a crisis that isn't perceived by others (including PD/ leadership) as a crisis per se. I feel like slowness to recognize crisis in a timely manner is one of the challenges (and one of my biggest failings as PD was not reaching out to our Black residents after George Floyd until one of them approached me); I was horrified by Floyd's murder, etc., but hadn't perceived the impact of my silence (and the silence of our white residency community) as compounding the crisis among our Black residents."*

In her TED talk on becoming "good-ish," Dolly Chugh points out that our pursuit of being viewed as a "good" person often gets in the way of becoming a better person (Chugh, 2018). She recommends letting go of the desire to be "good" and aiming instead for getting better or being "good-ish." Defensiveness in these moments of mistakes is so natural. Humility is harder, but, in the long run, more productive because we can learn from our mistakes. I'm still working on it.

Summary

When you realize a community crisis has begun, your residents will need support. You might not do or say the right thing, but stay in the game. Model grace, even if that sometimes takes the form of acknowledging the community's views of the medical system and forgiving yourself for not always having the right words. Be courageous enough to try to do what your residents and community need.

Table 6. Summary approach to community tragedies such as violent deaths or mass shootings	
Pre-Crisis	<ul><li>Know your risk management group</li><li>Recognize that a crisis is starting</li></ul>
Crisis	<ul><li>Take care of residents involved with the care of victims</li><li>Take care of yourself and acknowledge your own feelings</li><li>Reach out to all residents in your program</li><li>Engage risk management (if indicated)</li></ul>
Post-Crisis	<ul><li>Manage safety issues for residents if there is continued violence in the community</li><li>Realize that you aren't perfect and strive to be better</li><li>Look for opportunities to help the community heal</li></ul>

Citations

American Psychological Association. (2011). *Managing the Traumatic Stress of a Hurricane and Its Aftermath.* American Psychological Association. Retrieved September 11, 2023 from https://www.apa.org/topics/disasters-response/hurricane-stress

Association of American Medical Colleges. (2016). Faculty Diversity in U.S. Medical Schools: Progress and Gaps Coexist. *Analysis in Brief, 16*(6). https://www.aamc.org/media/8406/download?attachment

Bogel-Burroughs, N. (April 5, 2021). The Doctor Who Pronounced George Floyd Dead Says a Lack of Oxygen Was the Likely Cause. *The New York Times.* https://www.nytimes.com/2021/04/05/us/asphyxia.html

Public Health Foundation. (2024). *Welcome to CDC TRAIN.* Public Health Foundation. Retrieved January 15, 2024 from https://www.train.org/cdctrain/welcome.

Chugh, D. (October 2018). *How to Let Go of Being a "Good" Person – and Become a Better Person [Video]*. TED Conferences. https://www.ted.com/talks/dolly_chugh_how_to_let_go_of_being_a_good_person_and_become_a_better_person

Garrison, C. B. (2019). The Lonely Only: Physician Reflections on Race, Bias, and Residency Program Leadership. *Fam Med, 51*(1), 59-60. https://doi.org/10.22454/FamMed.2019.339526

Kalra, A., Reed, G. W., Puri, R., Majmundar, M., Kumar, A., Foley, J. D., Zala, H., Nasir, K., Kapadia, S. R., & Bhatt, D. L. (2022). Trend of Demographics of Cardiovascular Disease Fellows and Association Between Fellows and Program Director Race. *JACC: Advances, 1*(2), 100032. https://doi.org/doi:10.1016/j.jacadv.2022.100032

Livingston, I. (2022, October 4, 2022). What Made Hurricane Ian so Intense: By the Numbers. *The Washington Post*. https://www.washingtonpost.com/climate-environment/2022/10/04/hurricane-ian-statistics-deaths-winds-surge/

Nunley, L. (June 12, 2020). An Open Letter to my Colleagues. *The MedEd Blog*. https://transformational-times-blog.blogspot.com/2020/06/an-open-letter-to-my-colleagues.html

O'Connor, A. B., McGarry, K., Kisielewski, M., Catalanotti, J. S., Fletcher, K. E., Simmons, R., Zetkulic, M., & Finn, K. (2023). Internal Medicine Residency Program Director Awareness and Mitigation of Residents' Experiences of Bias and Discrimination. *Am J Med, 136*(7), 710-717.e713. https://doi.org/10.1016/j.amjmed.2023.03.003

Paetow, G., Scott, N., Panning, A., Hopkins, J., Aden, M., & Hart, D. (2023). Culinary Cultural Immersion: A Qualitative Analysis of Resident Knowledge, Attitudes, and Behavioral Changes Following a Brief Somali Cultural Immersion Experience. *AEM Educ Train, 7*(1), e10844. https://doi.org/10.1002/aet2.10844

Pallok, K., & Sekhri, S. (September 11, 2020). Racism is a Public Health Crisis: When Will We Decide It Matters? T*he MedEd Blog*. https://transformational-times-blog.blogspot.com/2020/09/racism-is-public-health-crisis-when.html

Patnaik, R., Attlassy, N., Davids, S., & Fletcher, K. E. (2022). A Reflection and Discussion Exercise on Racial Justice and Equity. *J Grad Med Educ, 14*(5), 554-560. https://doi.org/10.4300/jgme-d-21-00868.1

Ready.gov (2023a). *Build a Kit*. Department of Homeland Security. Retrieved October 30, 2023 from https://www.ready.gov/kit

Ready.gov (2023b). *Get Tech Ready*. Department of Homeland Security. Retrieved September 7, 2023 from https://www.Ready.gov/get-tech-ready

Reiley, D. G., Guldner, G. T., & Leinen, A. L. (2003). "You Are Commanded to Appear": The Subpoena and the Emergency Medicine Resident. *Ann Emerg Med, 42*(6), 843-846. https://doi.org/10.1016/s0196064403004451

Tanzilo, B. (February 2, 2023). Progress Report: ThriveOn Collaboration in the old King Drive Schuster's/Gimbels. *OnMilwaukee*. https://onmilwaukee.com/articles/thrive-on-progress-report

Whetstone, S. (2023). Reflections of a Black Program Director. *N Engl J Med, 388*(7), e18. https://doi.org/10.1056/NEJMpv2214871

CHAPTER 7

Leading Through a Pandemic

Alec B. O'Connor, MD, MPH

Danielle S. Wallace, MD

University of Rochester School of Medicine and Dentistry

In this chapter, the authors collectively revisit the early days of the pandemic, when moving through the unknown and a rapidly changing landscape required courage, gratitude, equanimity, and humility. While pandemics are rare, the principles described are applicable to other types of crisis. As the program director and chief resident of an internal medicine residency program, they recount that communication and coordination were key actions for their leadership team.

Introduction

Leading a residency program through a global pandemic is extraordinarily challenging. Program directors (PDs) must balance competing high-stakes priorities including the health, wellness, and learning of their residents while deploying them to work in potentially dangerous patient care settings; their own role as a healthcare provider and institutional leader; and the needs of patients and communities.

Early studies of the impact of COVID-19 on healthcare workers and studies from prior pandemics describe mental health effects including high levels of stress, depression, anxiety, insomnia, burnout, substance use, moral injury, and post-traumatic stress disorder (Fiest et al., 2021; Kisely et al., 2020; Myran et al., 2022; Preti et al., 2020; Schwartz et al., 2020). The younger, unmarried, early career physicians providing direct care to infected patients were at highest risk for adverse psychological outcomes (Fiest et al., 2021; Kisely et al., 2020). This describes many residents.

There are controllable factors that may help healthcare workers weather the stresses of a pandemic. For example, organizational support and confidence in the quality of just-in-time training and infection control measures have been found to be protective against adverse mental health effects in a pandemic (Preti et al., 2020). Clear, trusted communication from leaders can improve healthcare worker outcomes in a pandemic. This includes providing training and education about the infectious agent; transparency about required changes in job roles; enforcement of infection control procedures; providing for healthcare workers' basic needs (e.g., personal protective equipment [PPE], food, childcare, etc.); stress reduction and resilience training; access to and normalizing of the use of mental health care, peer and social support interventions; and the acknowledgement of and strategies to address moral injury (Kisely et al., 2020; Schwartz et al., 2020). Allowing staff some agency in directing their contributions, which would ideally be voluntary (though by necessity residents may have to contribute in ways they would rather not) and ensuring adequate and predictable time off are also helpful (Kisely et al., 2020). Finally, independent of pandemic times, residents' perception of and satisfaction with their program's leadership behavior is correlated with burnout and program satisfaction (Dyrbye et al., 2020).

Story #1: The COVID-19 Pandemic

In January 2020, the US media began to report a new virus producing SARS in Wuhan, China. The significance to our program was unclear initially. As more data emerged, including reports of COVID-19 producing community health crises in Europe (particularly in Italy), it became clear that COVID-19 would affect our residency in time. We anxiously followed news of the first US outbreak in Seattle and hospitals being overwhelmed in New York City.

On March 10, the first case of COVID-19 in a non-traveler was identified in our community (Rochester, NY), and our residency was immediately thrown into crisis as all schools closed and all community clinics shut down abruptly. A colleague called me that night, asking to cancel an elective for a resident scheduled to rotate with him the following morning in oncology clinic. Although my initial reaction was to doubt this was necessary, I deferred to his judgment. The following morning, we called an urgent meeting of program leadership to determine how and when to shut down "nonessential" rotations. This required us to define "essential rotations." Our chief residents, monitoring the situation through friends and colleagues around the country, helped us get past our own "Is this really happening??" reactions and helped us act more quickly and decisively.

Advice from the Literature and Practical Wisdom
Define the top priorities of the residency response

As described in Chapter 1, I can now see that our program entered the crisis phase March 10. For us, that meant mobilizing extra communication and rapidly adapting to the needs of multiple stakeholders. Our residency leadership team defined our early goals (Table 1), starting with protecting our residents' safety. Residents are a crucial part of the workforce, and their health ensures that patient care efforts can be sustained. Talking about our priorities with all stakeholders guided decision-making about resident deployment, new policies (e.g., how to protect the code team when they respond to a patient who might have COVID-19), and whether to have group events like noon conference. Communicating our priorities consistently and explicitly helped the residents understand our decisions, even if they weren't happy about them.

Table 1. Program priorities in pandemic crisis
• Top (short-term) priorities:
- Health and safety of residents
- Help medical center care for patients and the community
• Secondary (long-term) priorities:
- Resident education
- Resident wellness
- Resident morale

Meetings with leadership from different areas of the clinical enterprise focused on our residents' and patients' safety. I was ready to ask, "How do we ensure that the residents are safe while we . . . ?" in all crisis-focused meetings. Luckily, our medical center leadership shared our priorities, making it largely unnecessary for me to advocate for residents' safety. Not every PD in the country had that luxury.

Be prepared to digest, prioritize, and translate new and rapidly evolving information

Someone on the leadership team should be assigned to process the vast amount of incoming information. I felt compelled to be the one to learn and transmit as much as I could. For our residents, I focused both on practical information of immediate relevance and on the larger context. I focused on our residents' safety and practice, such as personal protective equipment (PPE), isolation protocols, and testing procedures created by our hospital. We directed our residents to our hospital's digital COVID-19 "landing page," which housed policies and practical videos (e.g., how to don and doff PPE, how to obtain a nasal swab for testing). I summarized and showed highlights of high-yield information during frequent, residency-wide meetings. In some cases, we invited local experts to address the residents directly (e.g., our hospital epidemiologist or ICU director).

> "I was compelled to learn as much as I could and to transmit that information to those who needed it."

I also focused on the bigger picture to put our local situation in the global context. I avidly read the *New York Times* and major medical journals. I followed the Johns Hopkins University Coronavirus Resource Center, the New York State health department, and our county health department websites. This helped the residents anticipate what might be coming next and helped us all manage our fears and anxiety.

At the same time, our residents had important information, concerns, and questions that needed to be heard. We welcomed their input and questions (directly to me, to our APDs and faculty, and to our chief residents) and sought the answers to questions when required. When we learned of a specific concern in a clinical setting, we immediately shared it with the leaders of that area (e.g., our ICU director, director of hospital medicine, or our residents' clinic sites). The leaders listened to the residents' concerns and addressed them if at all possible.

Your role as center of the program's communication just got bigger

A rapidly emerging deadly illness also creates extraordinary communication challenges locally and nationally that PDs must manage. The PD is the focal point (or bottleneck) of critical communication among a range of groups (Figure 1). During a pandemic, you will routinely communicate with program staff, residents and leaders from the GME office, the medical center, your department, and hospital units and clinics. Our program leadership participated in many emergency meetings with these groups, focused on creative problem solving. I shared the decisions and information with the residents.

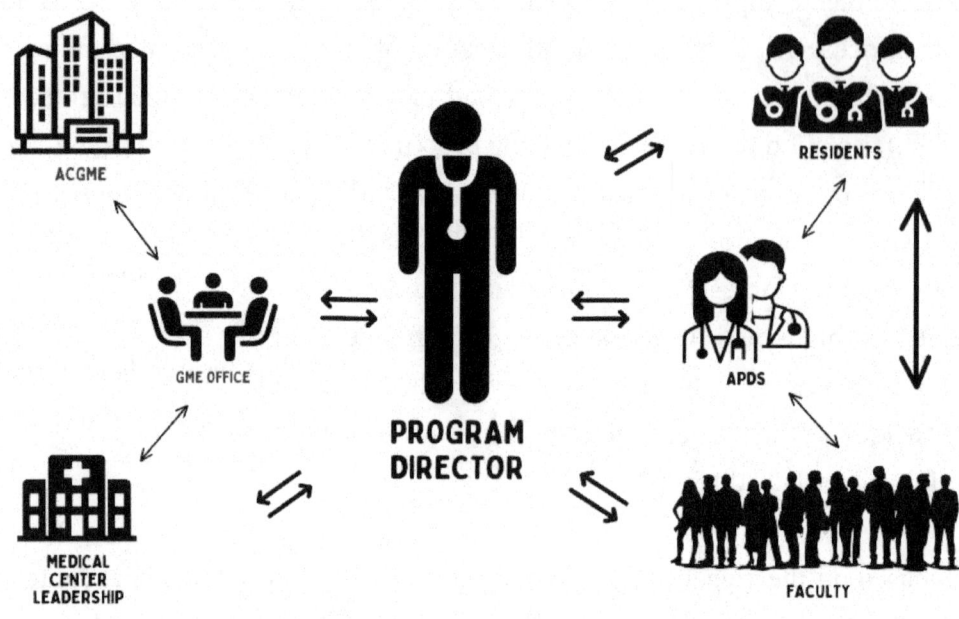

Figure 1. Program directors receive and share information from myriad sources during a crisis like a pandemic. The double arrows represent direct communication with the PD; the single arrows represent communication that does not directly involve the PD.

Frequent communication with your leadership team is essential

Intra-team communication must be frequent in the beginning of a pandemic. As the challenges related to the COVID-19 pandemic surged in Europe, our leadership team began discussing our local approach. Beginning in mid-March, we met at least daily, in addition to communicating often via text and emails. Much of this communication was reactive (e.g., a chief resident sharing that "our night residents need more help" or asking, "What should we tell the residents?"). Accumulating experience helped us better anticipate problems and issues. Our chief residents helped collect information, including the fears and concerns of the residents in various roles. They created solutions to emerging challenges. The "glacial" reserves that existed before the crisis (Chapter 1) were critical to our success: we trusted each other, had enough psychological safety to share fears and concerns, and had shared mental models for how to communicate with and support our residents.

Communicate clearly, consistently, frequently, and intentionally with residents

Bidirectional communication with residents was critical. We scheduled frequent (e.g., weekly, initially) program-wide Zoom meeting check-ins to share the latest information and provide updates (e.g., PPE availability, the latest policies and procedures, etc.). Some programs gave residents an opportunity to anonymously submit questions/concerns ahead of Zoom meetings, giving the leadership team a chance to gather information and formulate answers.

We also used email more frequently. We followed up resident Zoom meetings with detailed emailed minutes of the discussion to help keep all residents in the loop and to emphasize important "take home" points. We also sent email updates with new information and policy links as frequently as every other day between Zoom meetings. Other programs sent nightly emails, collating the most essential information for the residents so they did not have to sift through everything on their own. One program included a moment of levity at the end of each email, which the residents looked forward to reading. Each time we communicated with the residents, we encouraged them to reach out with any concerns or questions.

When we changed residents' schedules (which happened at an unprecedented rate), we started by providing the rationale and asking them to share their concerns. Residents had many reasonable questions about how their schedules and rotations were being affected. We answered as transparently as possible with the caveat that things could continue to change rapidly. When we didn't know something, we admitted it and tried to find the answer quickly.

The chief residents communicated with individual residents about schedule changes. Finding the best method and frequency for these updates was challenging. They needed to let the residents know about schedule adjustments quickly, but also wanted to avoid sending multiple emails because plans were changing so rapidly. The chief residents settled on communication when they had definitive updates. The chiefs also maintained an open-door policy for resident questions and concerns.

Connect with medical center leadership, even if you invite yourself

Our medical center created a "command center" with daily Zoom meetings that included updates about the number of COVID-19 cases locally, hospital capacity, testing capability, PPE stores, and the latest isolation, testing, and treatment guidelines. Our residency program was not initially invited to the command center meetings, but I asked to join and was able to participate in most of the meetings. While I rarely contributed to those discussions, knowing what our medical center leadership was facing, prioritizing, and concerned about helped me convey information to our residents that was in sync with messages sent broadly to all personnel. Occasionally, I would learn things that needed follow-up with command center stakeholders to keep us aligned.

It was critical for our program leadership to remain in contact with our Hospital Medicine Division chief, ICU director, and Dean of Graduate Medical Education (who is also our designated institutional official [DIO]) so we could support each other. Our DIO reached out to me frequently to see how our program and residents were doing. She created a small text group with PDs from the internal medicine, medicine-pediatrics, emergency medicine, anesthesia, and surgery programs, as these residency programs were most involved in adult inpatient coverage. During surges, we met as often as weekly and communicated regularly via text. Our DIO convened discussions about whether and when to convert our medical center to "emergency status" with the ACGME.

Building on our pre-existing relationship, the General Medicine Division chief and I communicated directly to coordinate clinic and residency program activities. As a result, we were able to implement precepted telehealth visits that allowed residents to provide continuity of care for their outpatients.

Identify and use external and pre-existing resources to inform decision-making
You may find non-standard resources helpful at the beginning of a pandemic because scientific evidence may be scarce. Critical preparedness information came from the Association of Program Directors in Internal Medicine (APDIM) listserv postings by John Choe, an APD at the University of Washington's internal medicine residency program in Seattle, where the first US outbreak affected a residency. John's posts contained frank descriptions of the challenges they were facing (learning to use PPE, struggling with inadequate testing, deploying residents into wards and ICUs full of COVID-19 patients). The posts also helped us prepare to fumble through the learning process with imperfection and without all the answers, but truly doing our best.

Pre-existing relationships through the APDIM "chief camp," among other connections, provided lines of communication between our chief residents and chief residents in other programs. These connections were invaluable sources of information and support. In particular, our chief residents helped our faculty leadership team understand the ramifications of various scheduling scenarios and played a pivotal role in protecting residents. Their benchmarking of what other programs were doing helped our program leadership make correct, but extremely difficult, decisions rapidly.

Plan for and attend to the myriad feelings of your residents

We saw a range of resident reactions to the pandemic. Many residents responded to the pandemic with a sense of duty, though some residents were terrified for both themselves and their families whether they were local or far away. Residents had ongoing concerns about bringing the deadly virus home to loved ones. Notably, a smaller number of residents seemed under-cautious and overly eager to put themselves at risk; some of these residents sacrificed their own wellness by contributing more than a reasonable amount to serve our patients' needs.

Being together frequently helped calm everyone. It reassured our residency community that we had an evolving plan, even if we didn't yet have all the answers. We were transparent about what we knew, what we were thinking about, what we were concerned about, and what we didn't know. I think transparency was generally appreciated by our residents. It helped build and maintain trust in our interventions and plans. Acknowledging residents' fears helped them feel less isolated. Meeting often and sharing our own concerns helped our residency community pull together. That helped all of us (myself included) cope with the extreme stress we were feeling.

Realize that these crises require nimble thinking

We literally "blew up" resident schedules when the pandemic became local, cancelling electives, ambulatory blocks, and all nonessential patient care activities. We prepared for anticipated surges, which didn't end up coming until later. This included contingency plans to have a group of residents "on standby" who were not scheduled for clinical activities, understanding they may be deployed to areas of need on short notice. We quickly converted teaching conferences to virtual formats, including morning report and noon conference. An unexpected upside of the virtual format was that more residents and faculty than ever before could participate in our conferences, including those on rotations during which they typically would not attend.

We explained the rationale for these changes (to protect residents and patients from viral spread while ensuring patient access for essential care), invited residents to share their concerns about our proposed plans, and, when possible, incorporated resident preferences and suggestions into our plans.

We encouraged, but didn't require, standby residents to join our virtual educational conferences, to pursue reading pertaining to electives they were missing, and to prepare for board exams. We expected that some residents would need that time to decompress emotionally and physically. Some programs designated an APD to create an individual learning plan for each resident on standby, promote accountability for time, and encourage individual residents to continue their education even as their experiential learning opportunities were curtailed. At some institutions, consult services offered "virtual rounds" and/or gave residents who were at home a list of recommended reading materials.

While much of the increased clinical work in the pandemic fell to internal medicine, family medicine, emergency medicine, and pediatrics, other specialties found ways to contribute. For example, in some institutions, anesthesia residents took on additional medical ICU responsibilities. Surgery residents took over the surgical ICUs to replace the anesthesia residents who had moved to the medical ICUs.

Some residency programs saw a sharp decrease in clinical work because they mainly saw patients in the clinics (e.g., dermatology), which were largely closed or because their inpatient work was predominantly elective (e.g., joint replacement surgeries in orthopedics). Some of those PDs had to create virtual visits and design supervision for such visits. They also had to move all their conferences to the virtual setting and design at-home educational experiences for their residents who were not needed in the hospital.

Allow/encourage residents to have a voice
As we redeployed residents into challenging work environments, including extra ICU and night float rotations, we surveyed our residents to identify individuals' preferences so we could align these extra experiences with learner preferences. For example, we had some residents who hated working overnight shifts and others who were especially uncomfortable working in the ICU. We tried but couldn't guarantee scheduling these residents in accordance with their preferences. Many residents volunteered to work extra nights and a handful volun-

teered to work extra ICU weeks. They were motivated by a combination of duty, interest in working with the sickest patients with a novel disease, and the opportunity to work directly with some of our remarkable critical care faculty and staff. We asked residents to provide input on how to best manage the challenges we were facing and improve/maximize their wellness within the constraints we faced.

Anticipate some professionalism issues
Colleagues elsewhere encountered difficulties with their residents. Some institutions gave "hazard pay" to non-physician staff and even faculty members while not extending this benefit to residents, which made some residents angry about the inequity. Advocating for the residents with institutional stakeholders is imperative for your relationship with them, even if you do not have direct control over resources such as resident pay. In one instance, a program was able to get moonlighting hours approved before the department asked the residency to provide more residents to cover inpatient services. This partially quelled resident dissatisfaction about not receiving hazard pay.

Other programs experienced unprofessional resident behavior in response to the stress of the pandemic. For example, some residents demanded extra allotments of PPE when it was still in short supply. A few residents simply refused to take care of patients with COVID-19. Some residents completing electives at home became angry when they had to do extra night work in overwhelmed ICUs. Such behavior frustrated PDs. There were times when it was impossible to give individual attention to these issues during the COVID-19 chaos. When there was adequate time and patience, empathic listening often worked to address emotions and arrive at a resolution. Of course, pivoting to firm policy adherence was necessary when it was not possible to accommodate individual exceptions, and ensuring that clearly unprofessional behavior was addressed was critical to maintaining a sense of fairness and justice among residents.

Help your leadership team help you
Starting early in the pandemic, I strove to ensure we were making the best possible decisions for the program. I leaned heavily on the program's leadership team to help me process the best available information, brainstorm possible solutions to new problems, and weigh the options available to us. I felt (and slept) better knowing that multiple people with multiple perspectives agreed with the high-stakes decisions we made.

I was fortunate to have a brilliant, supportive, creative, and proactively helpful leadership team willing, as individuals, to take responsibility for pieces of our program's response. APDs and chief residents could act with confidence and autonomy because of the glacial resources our leadership group had built up prior to facing the pandemic: valuable reserves of trust, shared mental models, and deep organizational knowledge which grew from pre-existing strong working relationships. For example, the ambulatory APD helped coordinate changes to ambulatory schedules and teaching. The inpatient APDs for our two hospitals communicated regularly with their hospital leadership while keeping me informed. I gave the chief residents full license to think creatively about the program structure, including the schedule and education. They viewed this ability to make decisions as a rare positive of the pandemic. The teamwork was essential.

Acknowledge resident frustration and provide morale support
With hindsight, some of what we did was certainly more intensive than necessary. Some residents sat at home for a month, waiting to be called in to work. We acknowledged their frustration with the uncertainty, constant change, and disruption to normal life. We worried about residents who were sheltering in place alone. We tried to support morale with surprise cookie deliveries, coordination of Zoom exercise and yoga classes, and holding a socially distanced graduation despite strict hospital policies. The residents often said they knew we were trying to do our best and appreciated the transparency.

Story #2: The Second Stage

By November of 2020, our residency had adjusted to the new "normal" of masking and social distancing. We had resumed electives, "nonessential" rotations, and our usual conferences, virtually or in hybrid form. We were in the post-crisis or recovery phase, and many residents were suffering from fatigue, frustration, and prolonged social isolation. In November, COVID-19 cases started rising exponentially, creating a crisis phase superimposed on the post-crisis phase. By mid-December, inpatient wards and ICUs were overwhelmed due to the severe COVID-19 surge (Figure 2). Our residency emergently doubled the internal medicine resident-staffed floor, ICU, and night teams at our main teaching hospital by pulling residents from nonessential rotations and essential rotations where the work could be done by advanced practice providers, fellows, or non-internal medicine residents.

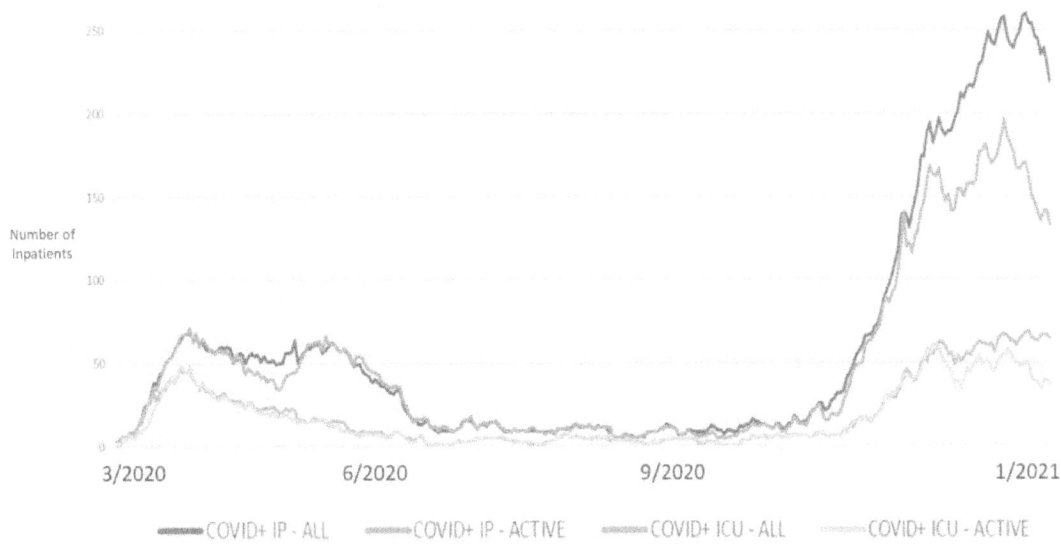

Figure 2. COVID-19 positive ("COVID+") inpatient ("IP") numbers in a 900-bed teaching hospital from March 2020 to January 2021. Discharging COVID+ patients after they no longer required hospitalization became a problem in the winter of 2020-2021, which exacerbated hospital overcrowding and staffing challenges (our hospital tracked the number of COVID+ patients who were "Active" and "Inactive" to understand how much of the hospital crowding related to discharge barriers).

Advice from the Literature and Practical Wisdom

Sometimes the post-crisis phase circles back into another crisis phase (Chapter 1) rather than into the hoped-for new pre-crisis phase. The November surge required us to re-engage our more frequent communications strategies and rethink using our residents to care for the influx of COVID-19 patients.

Look for untapped resources when a new crisis arises quickly

In addition to using residents on electives, look for other residency programs that can help and/or services that have advanced practice providers (APPs) who can temporarily take on more patient care. Because of the quick return to the crisis phase, we did not have residents at home in reserve, so we used all these strategies to get us through. For example, our cardiology and oncology rotations had APPs who took over the care of those services so that residents could move to floor teams focused on COVID-19 patient care. An affiliate hospital's family medicine residency took over our residents' inpatient care (along with APPs) so that our medicine residents could cover more patients in our main hospital. Some other programs' PDs increased admitting caps (still within the ACGME rules) and temporarily allowed resident teams to accept morning "rollover" admissions from the overnight hospitalist teams. At another site, PGY3 residents from electives were assigned to help on the COVID-19 hospitalist-only teams, but the residents still had nights and weekends off.

Clearly state and widely disseminate the rules that you will not break
Promise the residents that you will not violate core rules such as duty hour limits, supervision requirements, and caps. Having "will-not-violate" rules allows the residents to maintain basic expectations, even as other rules change. We shared our will-not-violate rules with hospital leadership as they looked to us to contribute to emergency care. Having proactively doubled the number of medicine residents in critical areas allowed us to say "We will not do this" in response to requests for our residents to do even more.

Focus on resident wellness
A sustained focus on wellness is necessary in a crisis that spans years. Resident wellness had been a concern throughout the pandemic. By the winter surge, some residents were experiencing fatigue, burnout, and reduced morale from prolonged isolation and diminishment of their usual supports.

You may have to take a stand with medical center leadership to preserve resident wellness. Social distancing rules became a big challenge for us because so much resident wellness flows from contact with each other. Our institution's social distancing rules around not providing food clashed with what we felt was important. For example, the residents needed to eat in the hospital, and we felt that forcing them to eat alone was not reasonable or feasible. We continued to provide lunches at conferences throughout the pandemic despite substantial resistance from medical center leadership. I found meetings with medical center leadership to advocate for bending these rules a very challenging part of the pandemic.

You should also create opportunities for fun. We tried little things. We highlighted people and successes on our program's Instagram account. We scheduled resident-run virtual game nights and book clubs. Other programs hosted fitness challenges and outdoor activities such as hikes.

You will likely have residents who need additional resources, and they may prefer to discuss such issues with a chief resident rather than faculty. We explicitly and repeatedly encouraged any resident who was feeling overwhelmed or burned out, experiencing mental health challenges, and/or just needing a break to let us know, and we'd help them get what they needed, including time off. A few residents needed to be taken off the extra COVID-19 teams.

Share gratitude and "small victories" generously

Take every available opportunity to publicly thank your residents for their bravery, adaptability, willingness to help in times of crisis, and their excellence. When you hear kudos from others such as faculty and nurses, share them broadly. For example, one of our nurses shared this praise about one of our residents' care of a dying patient, which I shared with our whole program:

> *"Meliora" stands for "ever better," and it is the pillar of Strong [Memorial Hospital] that makes our doctors and nurses stand out above the rest. In particular I want to recognize Chris for not only upholding those values but for being more than just a doctor for his patients. Chris was taking care of a patient that was steadily declining throughout the day and he made sure to keep the family informed while advocating for his patient's needs. This compassion carried on into the next day where Chris was by his patient's side when he needed him most by offering his support and comforting him while he was in his care. With everything going on during these times, it is hard to take the time to pay attention to the small details, but Chris made sure that he took the time to give the patient everything that he needed in his time of need. Thank you, Chris!*

The positive energy and "can do" spirit of our residents and chiefs kept me going during stress I never thought I would have to (or be able to) face.

Enter the post-crisis recovery phase

Eventually, the crisis phase of a pandemic will pass. The post-crisis or recovery phase may be the hardest to lead through because the disruptions of the crisis phase have worn people down and the initial "let's all pitch in" reactions fade. Recovery can be long and requires maintaining motivation and leading collaboratively (Geerts et al., 2021). A 2021 consensus guideline specific to the post-crisis recovery phase (Geerts et al., 2021) identified leadership "imperatives," several of which are pertinent to PDs (Table 2).

Table 2. Post-crisis leadership imperatives adapted to GME leadership teams (Geerts et al., 2021)
• Celebrate team and individual member successes
• Support well-being of team
• Prepare for future emergencies
• Reassess team priorities and provide inspiration to the team
• Maximize post-crisis team performance
• Revisit team activities that were paused or altered during the crisis
• Learn from the crisis and use that knowledge to innovate/improve team functioning
• Continue to communicate regularly with your team

Take stock when the crisis is over
Continue attending to the wellness of your leadership team and residents. Review the crisis with the leadership team. Identify points of pride and opportunities for improvement for future crises. Are there resources that you should ask for to help with recovery, such as additional funding for wellness? Ask your team what additional resources could make the team more effective in the next crisis, then ask departmental leadership for them. It may be difficult to revisit the crisis after living it for so long, but this is your chance to make your program stronger.

Usual conferences and long-standing policies from pre-pandemic times may have been altered or stopped. Make sure to take time to revisit what should be restarted and what is better in the new iteration. One program director realized that her chief residents had stopped doing morbidity and mortality conferences during the pandemic. Those needed to be restarted. Other changes seemed worth keeping, like having Zoom as an option for certain meetings. You may need to review and discard policies that were instituted to get through the surges.

Then take a deep breath, and remember to appreciate yourself for leading. It doesn't matter if you weren't perfect. You led. And if you won't say it to yourself, I will: "Well done. Thank you for your leadership."

Summary

Our residents and faculty stepped up heroically throughout the pandemic, selflessly throwing themselves into the most challenging situations. I will be forever grateful to our residents, staff, faculty, and chief residents for their incredible contributions.

Building and maintaining trust with residents was critical. We consistently shared what we knew and didn't know, shared our best projections of what to expect, and made it clear that we were extremely concerned about their safety while also trying to help our patients and community survive an unprecedented challenge. Whenever possible, we involved residents in identifying problems, creating solutions, and having a voice in how they were deployed. Honesty, humility, empathy, and availability within a supportive environment helped residents trust us and accept the changes and challenges of the COVID-19 crisis as well as could be hoped.

\multicolumn{2}{l}{Table 3. Concerns/priorities and questions to consider in a pandemic}	
Pre-Crisis	Build glacial resources • Do we have trust and shared mental models for program priorities in the leadership team? • Do we have trust and familiarity with the medical center, departmental and GME leadership? Monitor the transition • Is this a crisis?
Crisis	Protect the health of the residents (personnel resources) • Can we identify infected patients? • How can we limit residents' exposure to infected patients? • Do the residents know how to appropriately use PPE?

Crisis (cont.)	• How should residents respond to emergencies in infected patients (e.g., PPE don/doff delay)?
	
	Protect resident wellness
	
	• Are residents experiencing isolation, stress, fear, moral distress? If so, what can we do for them?
	
	Protect the health of patients
	
	• Is the workload per physician/APP safe?
	
	Coordinate with the medical center to optimize patient care and protect the residents
	
	• Who is representing the residents at the medical center level?
	
	• Are the residents an important part of the medical center response?
	
	• Is the medical center overly reliant upon the residents?
	
	• What are the residency rules that our program believes cannot be broken regardless of the severity of the situation?
	
	• What is the ACGME position on the use of residents during this crisis?
	
	• As policies change, how will they impact the residents?
	
	• How should the information from the medical center be managed for the residents?
	
	Communicate transparently and frequently with residents to optimize information and avoid panic
	
	• What information do the residents need now?
	   - About virus
	   - Navigation of system issues
	   - Changes to their schedules
	   - Other issues that directly impact them
	
	How can I best convey that we understand their concerns/sacrifices?
	   - How can we facilitate getting residents' input/concerns/ideas?
	   - Acknowledge some will need breaks and the program will support them through "unwellness"
	   - Gratitude for their hard work during stress/sacrifices

Crisis (cont.)	Communicate with other stakeholders • Does the medical center leadership know what we can and cannot provide? • Do the departmental leaders know our priorities? Adjust resident educational experience to the circumstances • How can we preserve the residents' educational experience? • What adjustments can be made to continue educational conferences? Build/preserve the program community • Can we bring people together during this crisis? • Are we adequately addressing resident concerns? • Are we celebrating small victories?
Post-Crisis	Tend to the emotional toll of the crisis • How is the leadership team coping? • How are the residents coping? • What can we do to rebuild our program community to promote healing? Show gratitude for what was accomplished • Are there notes of appreciation that can be shared widely? • Are there other accomplishments that we can celebrate? Review the program's crisis response • What did we learn about our weak spots? • Do we need additional resources to be prepared for next time or to recover?

Citations

Dyrbye, L. N., Leep Hunderfund, A. N., Winters, R. C., Moeschler, S. M., Vaa Stelling, B. E., Dozois, E. J., Satele, D. V., & West, C. P. (2020). The Relationship Between Residents' Perceptions of Residency Program Leadership Team Behaviors and Resident Burnout and Satisfaction. *Acad Med, 95*(9), 1428-1434. https://doi.org/10.1097/acm.0000000000003538

Fiest, K. M., Parsons Leigh, J., Krewulak, K. D., Plotnikoff, K. M., Kemp, L. G., Ng-Kamstra, J., & Stelfox, H. T. (2021). Experiences and Management of Physician Psychological Symptoms during Infectious Disease Outbreaks: A Rapid Review. *BMC Psychiatry, 21*(1), 91. https://doi.org/10.1186/s12888-021-03090-9

Geerts, J. (May 25, 2020). Our Approach to COVID-19 Won't Work as Well for a Second Wave. *The Globe and Mail.* https://www.theglobeandmail.com/opinion/article-our-current-approach-to-covid-19-wont-work-as-well-for-a-second-wave/

Geerts, J. M., Kinnair, D., Taheri, P., Abraham, A., Ahn, J., Atun, R., Barberia, L., Best, N. J., Dandona, R., Dhahri, A. A., Emilsson, L., Free, J. R., Gardam, M., Geerts, W. H., Ihekweazu, C., Johnson, S., Kooijman, A., Lafontaine, A. T., Leshem, E., . . . Bilodeau, M. (2021). Guidance for Health Care Leaders During the Recovery Stage of the COVID-19 Pandemic: A Consensus Statement. *JAMA Netw Open, 4*(7), e2120295. https://doi.org/10.1001/jamanetworkopen.2021.20295

Kisely, S., Warren, N., McMahon, L., Dalais, C., Henry, I., & Siskind, D. (2020). Occurrence, Prevention, and Management of the Psychological Effects of Emerging Virus Outbreaks on Healthcare Workers: Rapid Review and Meta-Analysis. *BMJ, 369*, m1642. https://doi.org/10.1136/bmj.m1642

Myran, D. T., Cantor, N., Rhodes, E., Pugliese, M., Hensel, J., Taljaard, M., Talarico, R., Garg, A. X., McArthur, E., Liu, C. W., Jeyakumar, N., Simon, C., McFadden, T., Gerin-Lajoie, C., Sood, M. M., & Tanuseputro, P. (2022). Physician Health Care Visits for Mental Health and Substance Use During the COVID-19 Pandemic in Ontario, Canada. *JAMA Netw Open, 5*(1), e2143160. https://doi.org/10.1001/jamanetworkopen.2021.43160

Preti, E., Di Mattei, V., Perego, G., Ferrari, F., Mazzetti, M., Taranto, P., Di Pierro, R., Madeddu, F., & Calati, R. (2020). The Psychological Impact of Epidemic and Pandemic Outbreaks on Healthcare Workers: Rapid Review of the Evidence. *Curr Psychiatry Rep, 22*(8), 43. https://doi.org/10.1007/s11920-020-01166-z

Schwartz, R., Sinskey, J. L., Anand, U., & Margolis, R. D. (2020). Addressing Postpandemic Clinician Mental Health : A Narrative Review and Conceptual Framework. *Ann Intern Med, 173*(12), 981-988. https://doi.org/10.7326/m20-4199

CHAPTER 8

Leading during Times of Legal Uncertainty: Legislative Disruption to Residency Training

Amy Domeyer-Klenske, MD

University of Wisconsin School of Medicine and Public Health

Kate Dielentheis, MD

Medical College of Wisconsin

In this chapter, the authors outline the challenges that arise when changing laws impact medical education policy and practice. They describe the courage, persistence, and innovation needed to face the implications for obstetrics/gynecology education after the June 24, 2022, Dobbs v. Jackson Women's Health Organization *(No. 19-1392, 597) US Supreme Court decision. In Wisconsin, programs had to restructure and relocate educational experiences. The authors used this legislative change as an opportunity to teach advocacy in real time while balancing sensitive political volatility.*

Introduction

The Supreme Court decision on *Dobbs v. Jackson Women's Health Organization* immediately changed the landscape for providing abortion care for patients in the US. In some states, it threatened physicians with criminal prosecution for providing medical standard of care services. As physicians and educators, we faced many challenging questions: How can we continue to provide appropriate care to patients needing these services? How do we avoid criminal liability for ourselves and our colleagues? How do we educate our trainees on required procedures that may now be illegal in our current area of practice? Unfortunately, on June 24, 2022, when this decision was released, there was no guidebook for managing this crisis.

Legislative interference with medical practice is not limited to abortion care or to the field of obstetrics/gynecology. Weinberger et al. laid out types of legislative interference, including laws that 1) prohibit physicians from having discussions with patients about risk factors that may affect their (or their family's) health, 2) require physicians to discuss practices that may not be necessary or appropriate according to the physician's best judgment, 3) require physicians to provide—and patients to receive—tests or interventions that are not evidence-based, and 4) limit the information that physicians can disclose to patients, to consultants in patient care, or both (Weinberger et al., 2012). See Table 1 for specific examples. *Dobbs v. Jackson Women's Health Organization* highlights the challenges of legislation interfering with medical education in addition to impacting the physician-patient relationship. Medical educators must be prepared to react to these policies to ensure access to evidence-based medical education.

Table 1. Examples of laws impacting the practitioner-patient relationship		
Law or Proposed Law	**Potential Impact on Practitioner-Patient Relationship**	**Current Status**
Florida Privacy of Firearm Owners ("Privacy of Firearm Owners," 2011)	Practitioners cannot ask patients about gun ownership	This provision was overturned in 2017 (Alvarez, 2017)
Palliative Care Information Act ("Palliative Care Information Act," 2011)	Practitioner must provide terminally ill patients with information about palliative care	In effect
Virginia House Bill 462 ("Amendment in the Nature of a Substitute," 2012)	Practitioner must provide a fetal ultrasound prior to an abortion	In effect
Alabama Vulnerable Child Compassion and Protection Act ("Alabama Vulnerable Child Compassion and Protection Act," 2022)	Practitioners are not allowed to provide or refer minors for gender-affirming care not consistent with their chromosomal sex	In effect

Story #1: A Totally New National Landscape for Reproductive Health Care

Following the Politico *leak of the impending US Supreme Court decision on* Dobbs v. Jackson Women's Health Organization *(Gerstein & Ward, 2022), our obstetrics/gynecology department was warned of the impending change, allowing us to prepare our clinical teams for the anticipated state of abortion care in Wisconsin when the decision was released. I recall a sense of impending doom amongst providers and trainees; we didn't know when or with complete certainty that the change would occur. Until that moment, many of us felt it was unimaginable the Supreme Court would completely strike down* Roe v. Wade, *immediately changing the practice of obstetrics and gynecology in our state. I remember sitting with colleagues and talking about how we would handle this as teachers, doctors, administrators, and mentors for colleagues and trainees, all of whom wanted to take action. Suddenly, we were overwhelmed, as abortion providers and gynecologists, by the need for action without guidance. We went from providing day-to-day abortion care to meeting with lawyers and trying to wrap our heads around the idea that we would cease providing care immediately when the decision became final.*

The weekend following the leak of the draft Dobbs v. Jackson Women's Health Organization *opinion coincided with our national American College of Obstetricians and Gynecologists (ACOG) conference. It was our first meeting in person since before the pandemic. We transitioned from what should have been a celebration of perseverance through the COVID-19 pandemic to yet another period of fear and uncertainty for our profession. Huddled in a hotel ballroom, we grieved, strategized, and prepared for the role we would play in the reproductive freedom culture wars.*

I was providing abortion care at Planned Parenthood on June 24, the day the decision was released. That day is one of those "seared-in-my-brain" experiences. I remember the husband of the last patient I cared for that day—aware of the precarious legality of the procedure—saying to me as I left the exam room, "This was a really big deal, wasn't it?" I nodded to him and walked out of the room. I saw the face of the center manager, who looked me in the eye and said, "It's done." We both started to cry. This decision impacted our trainees and us, not only in our jobs as physicians, but as individuals. We had to navigate caring for ourselves and each other in this time of monumental change both within our department and on a larger scale within our specialty.

In Wisconsin, an 1849 law bans abortion. It was nullified by Roe v. Wade (No. 70-18, 410 US 113) *but never repealed by the state legislature. When the* Dobbs v. Jackson Women's Health Organization *decision was released, our ability to provide and train our residents to provide abortion care was immediately halted until we could get further clarification from the state. This 1849 law not only bans the procedure, but imposes felony charges for physicians providing this service unless the life of the pregnant person is threatened. Many other states faced similar trigger laws. States where abortion remained a protected service ("haven" states) recognized the potential for an immediate increase in patients from banned states.*

We began conversations with our legal team about the clinical situations that would be affected by this law. Working with lawyers on institutional and state levels bridged the gap between the law and medicine. Furthermore, we collaborated with colleagues from institutions across the state to plan how we might provide legal abortion care under the maternal life exemption, attempting to find consensus despite the legal ambiguity.

Advice from the Literature and Practical Wisdom
Be prepared to navigate complex emotions about the political climate

Residency is already a challenging time, and residency leadership must help residents navigate the emotions from the many predictable challenges that they face. This is especially important in crisis. Even before the *Dobbs v. Jackson Women's Health Organization* decision, residents had complex feelings about learning and providing abortion care (Singer et al., 2015). Medically, the evidence regarding the importance of safe abortion care for patients has been well documented (National Academies of Sciences, 2018), but residents and attending physicians still carry their own personal feelings about pregnancy termination.

For many, the US Supreme Court decision represented a fierce strike on women's rights and bodily autonomy. Many residents and faculty struggled with anger, frustration, and hopelessness for themselves and their patients. Others celebrated the now legal preservation of fetal life. Because this viewpoint in our residency has been one in the minority, some residents have struggled to feel comfortable sharing their opinions and beliefs for fear of retribution. At a local listening session about experiences in the wake of the *Dobbs v. Jackson Women's Health Organization* decision, one anonymous contributor described feeling incredibly relieved that this decision halted abortion care in Wisconsin and further shared that this view had been met with negative feedback. Thus, the contributor did not feel safe sharing these feelings with others.

Leaders must help residents learn to talk among themselves about opposing viewpoints. It is increasingly important that trainees learn to engage in open, respectful, transparent dialogue that clarifies the tension between evidence-based medical care and personal values. Programs like Values Clarification help by encouraging residents to feel comfortable dealing with these complex reproductive health issues (Steinauer, 2015). This program provides a safe space to explore ideas, walking participants through challenging patient interactions and highlighting how personal beliefs and feelings affect our provision of care.

Keep residents informed
Regardless of the crisis, residents want information. When they do not hear from leadership, they become angry and fearful. After our institution's legal teams communicated the implications of the *Dobbs v. Jackson Women's Health Organization* decision, the residency leadership team emailed the residents to describe the legal reality in Wisconsin. They also offered reassurance that training experiences would be maintained in haven states and provided lists of resources for advocacy and mental health support. Later, we discussed with our residents how we as faculty have worked with colleagues around the state to develop guidelines to assist in medical decision-making.

In addition to communicating with the residents, we worked to craft a departmental message that was shared on our department website and social media outlets expressing support for the patient-physician relationship, evidence-based medical care in reproductive health, and a commitment to patients for excellence in care. Inviting institutional legal representation to discussions with trainees can also be valuable so that they can answer questions regarding the implications for the training program.

Develop a contingency plan for educational experiences
The ACGME requires specific clinical experiences for residents in each specialty. In obstetrics/gynecology, residents must have the opportunity to learn abortion care (ACGME, 2022). Our program would no longer be allowed to provide exposure to abortion care because of the legislative changes in Wisconsin. Therefore, we used connections through the Ryan Residency Program (The Kenneth J. Ryan Residency Training Program in Abortion & Family Planning, 2023) to begin the administrative work required for our residents to rotate at an outside institution. The Ryan Program works with residencies to provide resources and connection for robust abortion care training.

We worked with Rush University in Chicago, less than 100 miles away, to arrange visiting rotations in abortion training. To start, we decided that the third-year residents would get this experience. Third-year residents have developed their surgical skills and also have had experience with complex family planning conversations. This made them the ideal group to benefit from this intensive "away" rotation. Next, we drafted Program Letters of Agreement (PLAs), signed by both institutions. Our institution's legal team had to determine whether insurance for residents would cover their training at an outside institution performing procedures not legal in the state of their insurance. It did, as long as the procedures were legal in the state in which they occurred. This decision could vary between institutions, so consult your legal team. Residents had to obtain temporary/training licensure in Illinois before they could rotate there. In addition, they had to meet all administrative requirements of that institution's rotating resident policy, including TB skin testing and EPIC training. Our institution provided financial assistance for the residents' travel and accommodations. We communicate consistently with Rush's leadership, allowing us to maintain a strong working relationship, especially when unexpected issues arise.

Six months after the *Dobbs v. Jackson Women's Health Organization* decision, our first resident traveled from Milwaukee to Chicago for a two-week rotation; many have followed. The experience has been positive for our residents, but I was surprised to learn that it has also benefitted Rush's residents. They have appreciated the opportunity to learn about the delivery of obstetrics/gynecology care in a more restrictive environment like Wisconsin. They have also benefitted from the perspective of trainees from another institution about their residency experiences. The main downside for our residents is that what used to be an integrated, multi-year experience of learning about abortion care is now mostly limited to this intensive two-week-long rotation. Whether that is sufficient to achieve proficiency is to be determined.

Summary

New laws that impact patient care often impact education as well. Being honest with the residents and anticipating their fears are important characteristics of leadership in this type of crisis. Use national networks and regional resources to creatively address potential gaps in training. Work closely with your institution's legal team to design solutions.

Story #2: Engaging in Advocacy

Following the Politico *leak, we faced immediate changes in provision of care and education without the ability to proactively influence policy. We attempted to take responsibility with little power by controlling collaboration, physician messaging, and unity across the state with regards to physician-recommended reproductive healthcare. Physician leaders from the across the state came together to understand the 1849 law and to develop consensus on what abortion care could continue under the "maternal life" provision. This collaboration initially included practicing obstetrics/gynecology physicians who perform abortion care, those involved in legislative advocacy through the American College of Obstetricians and Gynecologists (ACOG), and maternal fetal medicine physicians through three major academic organizations in Wisconsin. Later, it grew to include physicians and lawyers at a variety of institutions state-wide. Thanks to a growing comfort with video conferencing, we held consensus discussions in the weeks following June 24, 2022. A self-identified leader prepared agendas and shared documents after meetings to ensure agreement. This consensus-building work gave confidence and comfort to those physicians who both educated trainees and provided life-saving care that they would not face criminal charges.*

Advice from the Literature and Practical Wisdom

Faculty who are facing a legally mandated change in medical practice may encounter trainees and colleagues who desire to advocate on behalf of their patients and their profession. In the wake of the Dobbs decision, there was a surge of interest in physician advocacy training and involvement. At that time, we had no standard advocacy curriculum.

The *Dobbs v. Jackson Women's Health Organization* decision was unique because of its immediate impact. Previously, when laws were proposed through our state's legislative process, we had the opportunity to influence the process. Two examples (described below) include a law that would have required written consent prior to a pelvic exam under anesthesia by a medical student (Opoien, 2021) and a law that would have prohibited Wisconsin state employees from providing abortion care (Mills, 2017). The second of these laws would have restricted residents at the University of Wisconsin from meeting ACGME accreditation requirements.

Develop your coalition

The first step in influencing policy is to build your coalition. For those new to advocacy work, identifying teammates can be as simple as querying your professional society or state medical society. Many of these organizations hire politically savvy lobbyists who advise members on legislative priorities, including which areas have potential to be legislative wins, and which are unlikely to yield meaningful change. Healthcare organizations working in a coalition to speak either with legislators or directly to the public through media interviews can have greater impact than a single individual or group.

For those areas in which policy change is unlikely—as was the case of abortion restrictions in Wisconsin—alternative courses of action might include efforts to influence public opinion through media or supporting candidates who might champion sound healthcare policy. However, be cautious! The Hatch Act limits federal employees (including those who work at Veterans Affairs sites) to participate in political activities while at work, on federal property, or in a government vehicle ("Hatch Act," 1939). In addition, federal employees cannot use their federal affiliation or title in political activities.

Get ahead of the issue and be ready to describe unintended educational consequences through a lens that politicians can support

Medical educators should remain informed about pending legislation that may impact provision of care and education in your specialty and foster relationships with legislators to help them understand how proposed policies could bolster or threaten medical education. In the scenario of the pelvic examination under anesthesia bill, we worked with our institution's government affairs team, the state medical society, and state specialty society to influence the legislation and inform legislators of the potential education impact of this policy.

Our written consent process had already included language about involvement of students as part of the surgical care team. While the legislation was pending, we made it explicit that a discussion about student involvement and examinations would occur during the consent process. Discussing this amongst the faculty allowed for a better understanding of how these conversations occurred in actual practice. We communicated back to legislators and our government affairs team that medical student involvement was already part of the standard consent. We reaffirmed our commitment to patient safety and autonomy while also avoiding new barriers to education and stigma about educating students on genital physical exam skills. This legislation has not passed the Wisconsin legislature at the time of this writing. Bills like this often resurface and require ongoing interaction with the legislators as interest in a particular proposal may ebb and flow.

In the case of the proposed legislation to prohibit University of Wisconsin employees from providing abortion care, a coalition of the state teaching hospitals plus our state ACOG chapter built relationships with legislators who were identified by professional lobbyists as key influencers on this policy. We communicated the significance of losing accreditation for our state university's obstetrics/gynecology program. Losing accreditation would have negatively impacted the ability to attract physicians to train in Wisconsin and would have affected providers choosing to continue their careers in Wisconsin. Once we put this into perspective, even lawmakers who generally supported anti-abortion legislation were opposed to this bill because they recognized the need to maintain educational programming in the state. We also developed relationships with the governor's office, which influenced decisions about vetoing related legislation, thereby preventing enactment of the myriad laws aimed at provision of abortion care and education prior to the *Dobbs v. Jackson Women's Health Organization* decision.

Engage trainees in advocacy

Many examples of advocacy curricula in residencies exist. A systematic review noted that the ACGME requirements, institutional support, and having experienced faculty facilitated the adoption of such curricula (Howell et al., 2019). When facing a difficult or inequitable policy situation, start an advocacy curriculum. Perhaps the *Dobbs v. Jackson Women's Health Organization* decision will prove to be such a facilitator, but any local or national issue could be a motivator to get started. For example, a psychiatry program initiated an advocacy elective to enable their residents to work on social determinants of mental health (Mathias et al., 2023). Many of our residents want to be involved in legislative advocacy on behalf of their patients, not only related to abortion care but other pressing issues like maternal morbidity and mortality, racial disparities in access to care, and others. The physician voice is strong, and residents recognize their power to help change minds as well as laws. We support residents who want to be involved in advocacy through our state medical society (The Wisconsin Medical Society) and specialty groups like ACOG. Our residents find meaning in advocating for their patients. In taking a more global view about the responsibility of a physician, programs can encourage and mentor residents to be involved in their community in a way that is consistent with their own personal values (Table 2).

Table 2. Possible community involvement activities
• Involvement in local and regional societies where local issues are addressed
• Attendance at community events such as film festivals featuring movies from or about the local community
• Protected time to do community-based activities

An advocacy curriculum does not have to be composed of lectures or didactics. It could be a living lab where trainees experience firsthand engagement in advocacy for effective health policy. We teach our residents to build relationships with specialty society lobbyists, media, government affairs teams, and the state medical society. For example, residents can participate in Wisconsin's annual Doctor Day, a legislative/lobbying conference sponsored by the state medical society. During Doctor Day, faculty and trainees learn advocacy skills before meeting with state legislators to advocate for legislative priorities. By fostering relationships for residents within our state specialty society, they met with political candidates, had opportunities to testify for important health legislation, and got access to media events and press conferences.

Craft a media message in tandem with communications staff

In my first interview with a print journalist about abortion care in Wisconsin, I felt nervous and unprepared. As physicians, we are trained to maintain patient privacy, which leads to fear about publicly describing our daily work. Yet during that interview, I recognized the importance of our conversation. With so much misinformation about reproductive healthcare, doctors must share the impact of restrictive abortion laws on patients and the various circumstances that lead to seeking such care. We can maintain privacy and also be part of the conversation that gives humanity and nuance to this politically charged dichotomy.

Regardless of the topic, physicians should work with the media to share health information with the public. Media relations programs through specialty societies or institutions can connect physicians with media requests. Institutions vary on their policies regarding physicians using their academic affiliation; therefore, determine institutional guidelines up front. Inform trainees who are interested in advocacy work of these guidelines, including how they apply to social media posts. Intentionally teaching residents how to have healthy relationships with the media will allow trainees to recognize the positive impact they can have through advocacy.

It is important that program directors, faculty, and trainees engage their institutional government affairs and communications staff if hoping to publicly advocate on behalf of the institution. Those hoping to advocate must be aware of institutional policies on public statements. If an institution chooses not to publicly support a legislative strategy or a media message, faculty and trainees could consider advocating as individuals or within their state medical or professional society as outlined below. Additionally, advocates should be discouraged from using work email for personal communications regarding advocacy that is not on behalf of their organization.

Story #3: The Impact on Residents of Practicing Medicine in Environments with Volatile Health Policies

I was sitting on the labor and delivery unit with one of our residents following the Dobbs v. Jackson Women's Health Organization *decision. We were discussing a patient scenario warranting use of the maternal life exemption. The common refrain of "How sick is sick enough?" had echoed in my own brain as I tried to balance caring for sometimes critically ill patients in our tertiary care center with the legal uncertainty created by the 1849 abortion ban. The resident looked right at me and said, "Well, we won't really find out until one of us goes to jail."*

I felt sick. I remembered my own residency: the fatigue from late-night studying and too-early alarms, the groan of my feet after an 80-hour week in the hospital. I couldn't imagine adding a fear of being arrested for practicing evidence-based medicine. As educators, we want our trainees to feel safe and have nurturing environments in which they can thrive. In this moment of uncertainty, however, I felt we might be failing them.

Advice from the Literature and Practical Wisdom
Provide clarity and reassurance to your trainees, to the extent possible

We discussed with faculty and residents the consensus guidelines about interpretation of the 1849 law. However, medical consensus is not legal consensus, so the risk for legal action is still a factor, especially with regard to trainee involvement. Attending physicians must have one-on-one discussions with residents about resident discomfort with any aspect of patient care. That includes giving trainees the opportunity to talk about their personal values with respect to abortion care as well as evidence-based medicine regarding care for pregnant persons and the data we have regarding abortion care.

For decisions about abortion, we first describe our rationale for why we think that this is the optimal/safest course of action. We give the resident the option of stepping away from the patient's care to prevent legal risk to the resident. Then, we give the resident space to decide for themselves. Our experience is that they want to provide the best care, too, and usually choose to continue as part of the team. When the patient cannot receive the care that they want in our state (for example, a severe fetal anomaly that does not threaten the life of the mother), we teach the residents how to help the patient get to a state in which they can receive the care they desire.

Strategize about recruiting interns (and retaining faculty) in a difficult political climate
There is significant concern about recruitment and retention of physicians in states like Wisconsin, given the political climate (Hoffman, 2022; Pollard, 2022). Obstetrics/gynecology residency applicants are keenly aware of the importance of abortion training, and we are seeing a decrease in applications to programs in states with laws limiting or banning abortion care (Murphy, 2023). A recent medical student told me, "There's no way that I would train in Wisconsin—I came to medical school to be an obstetrician/gynecologist and ultimately practice reproductive healthcare abroad. There's no way that I will get adequate training in a state like Wisconsin, so I wouldn't even consider staying." We hope to recruit residents to our program who will advocate for reproductive healthcare in Wisconsin. Many programs, however, continue to struggle as the need for training exceeds the capacity. We will likely see the ramifications for years to come, even if state law changes to enable training in abortion care in the near future.

I've been asked during interviews about my own experience as an abortion provider, and why I don't leave Wisconsin for another state. I tell them that right now, I'm needed here—the patients of Wisconsin need me to continue to advocate for them, fight for their rights, and be here to take care of them the second we can provide abortion care to all patients again. I tell them, "Going to another state is like pouring water on a house that isn't on fire. I don't want to go into the burning house, but if you don't go into the burning house, you aren't doing anything helpful. You've got to fight the fire, and the fire is HERE."

Many residents may finish their training and choose to leave states like Wisconsin and practice in a state where abortion is not criminalized, in part to simply remove the constant duress of decision-making. We fear the future of medicine in our state and recognize that the disparities in care for patients will likely widen as graduating residents (i.e., potential faculty members) choose to leave states like Wisconsin to avoid prosecution for comprehensive, full-spectrum obstetrics and gynecology care.

Re-imagine medical education post–*Dobbs v. Jackson Women's Health Organization*

For obstetrics/gynecology, graduation and certification requirements include comprehensive reproductive healthcare training in contraception and pregnancy termination. Residents are tasked with accomplishing at least 20 dilation and curettages (D&Cs) for miscarriage management or abortion. Arguably, more than 20 procedures are necessary to manage complex situations of post-abortion hemorrhage or infection. For this reason, residents worry about the adequacy of training they receive in abortion care and their ability to be an independent practitioner upon graduating.

Residents who want to practice in low-resource settings (e.g., rural communities) want to be able to handle a variety of challenging situations independently. We used three strategies to ensure adequate training. First, we collaborated with Rush University to arrange two-to-four-week rotations, in which our residents perform first and second trimester abortion procedures full-time. Second, we developed simulation for D&Cs, dilation and evacuations, post-abortion hemorrhage, and post-abortion IUD placement through a grant from the Association of Professors of Gynecology and Obstetrics. The goal is to practice skills during simulation that can be translated quickly during a more concentrated experience outside our institution. Third, we instituted an outpatient gynecology rotation which exposes residents to a higher likelihood of involvement in miscarriage management, including skills on options counseling and office manual vacuum aspiration. We hope this combination of experiences will give our graduates confidence in their future practice, regardless of the setting.

Summary

The *Dobbs v. Jackson Women's Health Organization* decision resulted in resident fear about patient care, graduating with potential education deficits, and the possibility of prosecution in an uncertain legal environment. The decision also required quick thinking about new approaches to abortion education and stimulated opportunities for advocacy education and discussion. We recommend using open communication with the residents as a group and in personal interactions to help address fears. Use creativity and collaboration to provide necessary experiences. Finally, take advantage of the opportunity to motivate residents to learn advocacy skills that are consistent with their personal values.

	Table 3. Summary approach to training in the setting of legal uncertainty
Pre-Crisis	<ul><li>Establish psychological safety within the leadership group</li><li>Establish psychological safety among the residents by preparing them to navigate differing viewpoints on a range of issues</li><li>Have someone on the leadership team be active in state medical societies to enable ad hoc working groups to be established quickly in a future crisis</li></ul>
Crisis	<ul><li>Manage the emotions of residents and leadership team</li><li>Be prepared for differing viewpoints and make a safe space for expressing them</li><li>Communicate with the residents as information and plans become available</li><li>Bring in the institutional legal team for clarification, if appropriate</li><li>Develop a plan for required educational activities if they cannot be accomplished in your state</li><li>In patient cases with legal uncertainty, have individual discussions with involved residents and allow them to decide on their own involvement</li><li>Use connections with the state medical societies to coordinate efforts across affected training programs</li></ul>
Post-Crisis	<ul><li>Identify new educational opportunities (e.g., implementing an advocacy curriculum)</li><li>Assess the efficacy of new educational activities</li><li>Mitigate the impact of the legislation on resident and faculty recruitment and retention</li></ul>

Citations

Alabama Vulnerable Child Compassion and Protection Act, Act No. 2022-289. Legislature of Alabama (2022). https://www.billtrack50.com/BillDetail/1446900

Alvarez, L. (February 16, 2017). Florida Doctors May Discuss Guns With Patients, Court Rules. *The New York Times.* https://www.nytimes.com/2017/02/16/us/florida-doctors-discuss-guns-with-patients-court.html?_r=0

Amendment in the Nature of a Substitute, House Bill No. 462, General Assembly of Virginia (2012). https://lis.virginia.gov/cgi-bin/legp604.exe?121+ful+HB462H1

Accrediation Council for Graduate Medical Education. (2022). *ACGME Program Requirements for Graduate Medical Education in Obstetrics and Gynecology.* https://www.acgme.org/globalassets/pfassets/programrequirements/220_obstetricsandgynecology_2022v2.pdf

Gerstein, J., & Ward, A. (May 3, 2022). Supreme Court Has Voted to Overturn Abortion Rights, Draft Opinion Shows. *Politico.* https://www.politico.com/news/2022/05/02/supreme-court-abortion-draft-opinion-00029473

Hatch Act, 5 U.S. Code § 7323 76th United States Congress, 7323 Cong. Rec. (1939). https://osc.gov/Services/Pages/HatchAct.aspx

Hoffman, J. (October 27, 2022). OB-GYN Residency Programs Face Tough Choice on Abortion Training. *The New York Times.* https://www.nytimes.com/2022/10/27/health/abortion-training-residency-programs.html

Howell, B. A., Kristal, R. B., Whitmire, L. R., Gentry, M., Rabin, T. L., & Rosenbaum, J. (2019). A Systematic Review of Advocacy Curricula in Graduate Medical Education. *J Gen Intern Med, 34*(11), 2592-2601. https://doi.org/10.1007/s11606-019-05184-3

Mathias, C. W., Sandoval, J. F., & Noble, S. E. (2023). Reflections on Piloting a Health Policy and Advocacy Curriculum for Psychiatry Residents. *Acad Psychiatry,* 1-5. https://doi.org/10.1007/s40596-023-01781-x

Mills, S. (2017, July 18, 2017). Medical Groups: Wisconsin Abortion Bill Would Jeopardize Doctor Training. *Wisconsin Public Radio.* https://www.wpr.org/medical-groups-wisconsin-abortion-bill-would-jeopardize-doctor-training

Murphy, B. (2023). *After Dobbs, M4s Face Stark Reality when Applying for Residency.* American Medical Association. Retrieved November 2nd, 2023 from https://www.ama-assn.org/medical-students/preparing-residency/after-dobbs-m4s-face-stark-reality-when-applying-residency

National Academies of Sciences, Engineering, and Medicine. (2018). *The Safety and Quality of Abortion Care in the United States.*

Opoien, J. (2021, July 29, 2021). Wisconsin Lawmakers Renew Effort to Require Informed Consent for Pelvic Exams under Anesthesia. *The Cap Times.* https://captimes.com/news/local/govt-and-politics/election-matters/wisconsin-lawmakers-renew-effort-to-require-informed-consent-for-pelvic-exams-under-anesthesia/article_fffd891f-8369-5772-86b0-271b18b7eed0.html

Palliative Care Information Act, Public Health Law Section 2997-c, New York Department of Health (2011). https://www.health.ny.gov/professionals/patients/patient_rights/palliative_care/information_act.htm

Pollard, J. (2022, October 19, 2022). Abortion Access Looms over Medical Residency Applications. *AP News.* https://apnews.com/article/abortion-health-business-education-family-medicine-3fbeef4338fb-dcaf48f4f133055c9f78

Privacy of Firearm Owners, CS/CS/HB 155, Florida House of Representatives (2011). https://www.myfloridahouse.gov/sections/Bills/billsdetail.aspx?BillId=44993

Singer, J., Fiascone, S., Huber, W. J., III, Hunter, T. C., & Sperling, J. (2015). Four Residents' Narratives on Abortion Training: A Residency Climate of Reflection, Support, and Mutual Respect. *Obstetrics & Gynecology, 126*(1). https://journals.lww.com/greenjournal/fulltext/2015/07000/four_residents__narratives_on_abortion_training__a.9.aspx

Steinauer, J. (2015). *When Abortion Is Not Available.* Innovating Education in Reproductive Health. Retrieved May 9, 2023 from https://www.innovating-education.org/course/when-abortion-is-not-available/

The Kenneth J. Ryan Residency Training Program in Abortion & Family Planning. (2023). *The Ryan Residency Training Program is a national initiative to integrate and enhance family planning training for obstetrics and gynecology residents.* The Kenneth J. Ryan Residency Training Program in Abortion & Family Planning Retrieved November 2, 2023, from https://ryanprogram.org/

Weinberger, S. E., Lawrence, H. C., 3rd, Henley, D. E., Alden, E. R., & Hoyt, D. B. (2012). Legislative Interference with the Patient-Physician Relationship. *N Engl J Med, 367*(16), 1557-1559. https://doi.org/10.1056/NEJMsb1209858

CHAPTER 9

Leading through a Personal Crisis:
An Unexpected Serious Illness in the Program Director's Family

Aimee K. Zaas, MD, MPH

Duke University School of Medicine

In this chapter, Dr. Zaas takes us on the very personal journey of leading a residency program (and a family) while navigating a personal crisis: her husband's leukemia diagnosis and treatment. We are reminded that leaders experience their own crises that do not directly involve their constituents, and leading through such crises requires different decisions and leadership skills than other crises. She describes her own growth as a leader committed to honesty, transparency, stability, and family/work balance. She shares her learned wisdom about accepting help and advice, the unexpected joy of sharing her experience in real time through a blog, the outpouring of support from a diverse group of people, and the hard decisions about how to maintain stability in her program and her family.

Introduction

As program director, you are often seen as a source of stability during a crisis. While you are unlikely an expert in whatever led to the crisis, your role and relationships with residents require you to step in, speak up, and work with other leaders to provide a path forward. What happens if the crisis involves you? Leading through a crisis that is personal requires a different set of skills and active decisions about your comfort with personal transparency and reliance on your team.

A short-term crisis may require these skills and attributes to be employed once; however, an extended event will require adapting crisis management over time. When the crisis involves your family, the acuity of the term "balance" can really strike home, requiring delegation of work responsibilities to others, accepting help from those you may have a supervisory relationship with, and even dealing with conflicting emotions when it is "easier" to be in your professional life than it is to be in your personal life. Depending on the duration of the crisis, you may find yourself adapting your roles and identity over time.

Our Story

Our story begins with an unexpected, high-impact medical event that required immediate action: my husband Dave, a well-known and prominent physician in the same hospital where I am residency program director, was diagnosed with acute myeloid leukemia just as recruitment season was ending. My internal medicine residency program is large (160 residents), and I have five associate program directors (APDs) on my team. At the time, our two sons were in middle school, and the residents knew them quite well as they had "grown up" in the program. They were classmates and friends with many of our colleagues' children as well.

The first 48-72 hours after diagnosis were a complete whirlwind, and, as a recovering intern myself, I entered "checkbox mode," a reflexive and comforting state of being: get the grandparents into town to help with childcare, tell the kids, inform family and friends, get coverage for Dave's clinical activities and administrative work, tell our team members, and somehow communicate both seriousness and stability to the residents. We opted to use a blog to update our family and friends. Dave's first blog entry really showcased his mindset, as well as his thoughts on the role of the healthy partner/decision-maker (me), particularly one with medical knowledge.

> **Dave's first blog entry defined my role in his illness:**
> "... I always thought if I was ever a patient I would want to know everything, but right now I just want to do what I am told and do it better than anyone else. I do not want to know my test results, prognosis or research different treatment options. I am extremely fortunate that Aimee can be that advocate on my behalf. I just want to focus on getting out of bed every day and doing what I can to stay strong..."

As the designated decision-maker for his care (as physicians, we are all familiar with the "wife with the notebook" in the patient's room), my main tasks were 1) meeting with the care team for treatment plans, 2) delegating my work to colleagues, and 3) informing the residents what was happening. Dave's imminent admission to the hematologic malignancy service, where residents are the primary caregivers, necessitated immediate action.

We planned a meeting to tell the residents. When they assembled in the usual conference room for the meeting, I was seated, facing them. David was behind me, wearing a mask way before masking was a thing, and our beloved palliative care attending doctor sat next to us. I remember that I was careful to say clearly that we had learned the night before that David had acute myelogenous leukemia and would be admitted that morning to the inpatient service. I specifically noted that we were asked if we wanted a resident to take care of him, to which we said, "Don't you know us?" That drew some nervous laughter. I remember expressing uncertainty about what the next weeks would entail, but that the rest of the leadership team would be running the program. The fellowship letters were written, and the grandparents had already arrived. I also assured them that it was okay to text or email during this time, in hopes of pre-answering any question about what was "proper" or "right." The post-meeting minutes were a blur of hugs and tears, and we left to proceed with the admission while the leadership team stayed to allow residents to debrief as needed.

The announcement of my husband's illness was the start of a nine-month leadership journey as he underwent treatment, bone marrow transplant, and dealt with post-transplant complications before returning to work, ultimately disease-free. Shortly after the diagnosis, we made the decision to seek care for Dave at the hospital where we trained so that he could participate in a clinical trial. I felt this decision would also relieve the residents of the responsibility of caring for their PD's husband and defuse one challenge of this crisis.

Should you ever wonder or doubt what kind of impact a program director can have in the lives of residents, Dave and I actually stayed in the home of our former program director (first, just me while Dave was hospitalized, and then both of us during the five months of his outpatient bone marrow transplant).

> **My blog entry from our arrival in Baltimore highlighted the depth of our support system:**
> *"As a current program director, it is really special to me that during the worst time of our lives, here I am, staying at my residency program director's house . . ."*

Throughout the journey, we worked to maintain the core values we outlined in the early conversation with the residents, including honesty and transparency, ensuring stability, and attempting to showcase the ever-elusive "balance" between work life and home life.

Advice from the Literature and Practical Wisdom

Plan the disclosure

First, we decided to hold an in-person emergency meeting of the residents where *together* Dave and I could tell them directly what was happening. We made a quick plan with a trusted colleague before the disclosure, similar perhaps to how one might plan to approach a family meeting to deliver challenging news. It made sense to consider several other decision points before the meeting.

First, we set goals for the meeting (Table 1). We focused on the trust and support that can be harnessed when we are transparent and share in profoundly vulnerable times. We also wanted to show stability and to reassure the residents that their careers and needs would be supported by the leadership team even as I stepped back temporarily. Finally, we hoped to illustrate that it is both accepted and expected to step back from work when a family crisis occurs (family > work). As described below, our decisions about how to construct the meeting tied directly to these goals.

Table 1. Meeting Goals
1. Show honesty
2. Show transparency, to the extent possible given clinical unknowns
3. Convey information
4. Convey trust in residents
5. Convey trust in the leadership team and stability for the program/residents
6. Convey that it is okay to have family be more important than work

Next, we decided who else would need to be present for the disclosure. We included our residency leadership team (support/stability/team): the four chief residents, five APDs, program coordinator, and other key program staff. We also had the Chair of Medicine attend (support/stability/team). She was very involved in the residency program, and we wanted the residents to know that the departmental leadership would support them through the journey. A key residency program tenet is to seek opportunities that are bigger than just oneself. The Chair of Medicine's presence also demonstrated the department's unwavering support for both the residents and us. This was such a big moment in our lives, we wanted to make sure that the residents felt seen. We also included a beloved palliative medicine attending physician who was already well known to the residents. It was important to us that he be available after Dave and I left the meeting to provide additional support. We decided ahead of time that I would do most of the talking to show honesty, transparency, and trust, but with my husband present in the room to also show the importance of prioritizing family.

Take stock of the decisions that need to be made

You will likely be unable to think of everything that needs to be decided or handed off, but try to outline the major decisions that will allow you to step away, at least temporarily. I had a series of practical decisions to make at this juncture, including whether to take a formal leave of absence (LOA), how to divest from upcoming inpatient ward attending duties, and how to delegate program-level responsibilities to my team. These mirror what attorney and trauma-informed leadership coach Katharine Manning states are the five principles of trauma-informed "grief leadership": share information, model healthy grieving, provide necessary resources, inspire, and take care of yourself (Manning, 2022).

Decide if you need to take a formal LOA

Deciding to take a LOA is personal and might change as the situation evolves. The decision depends on what you, your family, and your person in crisis need and may include financial pressures. My considerations included my children, who were old enough to have some self-sufficiency; in-laws who dropped everything to stay with my children; an established au pair who knew our family; and a deep network of friends who provided everything from rides to soccer to lunch-meal trains. In essence, others took over our family's independent activities of daily living. Because of this support, I could choose based on what I needed.

I decided not to take a formal LOA. I found that having some work to do was a sanity saver. Working (especially administrative tasks) allowed me to feel some sense of normalcy and control over some aspect of my life. As soon as we learned of the diagnosis, I met with my chair, who asked me what I needed to get through the crisis and then supported my decision by helping me give away some, but not all, of my PD responsibilities. She wanted me to focus on Dave, and she wanted me to do it on my terms. If I had wanted to take a LOA, she would have supported that decision, too. She calmly assured me at the end of the meeting that we would figure it out and make adjustments to my plan if needed.

Delegate some (or all) of your leadership work

Think about your leadership team objectively and make an assessment about how you will delegate responsibilities. Is there a long-standing APD who possesses deep organizational knowledge of the program and has a shared mental model of the program that is consistent with yours? Does that person have your trust and the trust of the other APDs? Maybe you would consider handing the program off to that person. Is there an APD who has time or something they can give up temporarily to accommodate increased program responsibilities? If there is no one person, tasks could be divided between APDs (and even the chief residents). This is a good time to assess the glacial resources described in Chapter 1 to determine to whom and how you will hand off responsibilities.

One of my senior APDs ran intern recruitment, which had just ended. The chair and I agreed he was the best option, and she reassigned his upcoming clinical work and increased his compensation so he could take on additional responsibilities. I handed off the day-to-day running of the program to him, including reviewing rotation evaluations, ensuring that my advisees got the meetings they needed, planning new intern orientation with the program coordinator, meeting regularly with the chief residents, and leading program meetings when I was away. He also took care of the unexpected minor dramas that occur in any program and made sure that the leadership group was visible to the residents.

For some APDs, taking on a bigger leadership role may be an important growth opportunity. Others may not aspire to more leadership but are still willing to help. One PD colleague was awarded a short sabbatical. Her most senior APD stepped into the PD role and thrived. That stint as the "stand-in PD" brought her increased respect and attention from departmental leadership and led to a coveted award nomination. Have enough awareness of your local environment to appropriately delegate tasks and responsibilities. Once you delegate, don't meddle.

> *"Have enough awareness of your local environment to appropriately delegate tasks and responsibilities. Once you delegate, don't meddle."*

My chair and I designed a schedule in which I would work in person most Mondays through Wednesdays and be away with Dave Thursdays through Sundays, although this varied with the treatment schedules, kids' activities, and a few high-profile work events like resident graduation. While being prescriptive about the schedule may seem like "micromanaging," the stability and predictability helped both our family and the residency maintain a sense of normalcy as we moved from early (phrenetic) crisis mode to calmer times of Dave's treatment and ongoing care. At all points, be clear about when you're available, who oversees what, and what you will still be doing.

Navigate getting medical care that may involve your trainees

As we are medical professionals, a personal or family illness most likely will play out in our own healthcare system. As our story moved quickly to another hospital due to clinical trial availability, we did not have to wrestle with the decisions about having "my" residents care for my husband, except for when they did the initial brief admission prior to transfer. Depending on the care needed, this decision may be dictated by hospital structure. It is important to be thoughtful and transparent about the role of housestaff in the care of a family member, given the power differential that exists between the PD (or any faculty member) and the housestaff. A poor clinical outcome could be especially difficult to navigate. Should you decide not to have housestaff take care of your loved one, be explicit about how you weighed your trust in their care versus your concern for their well-being in such a high pressure situation.

Make accommodations to your clinical (and other non-PD) work

Ask yourself if it is realistic to do clinical work during the crisis. You may not be able to effectively concentrate on the patients to the extent that they need/deserve. In my case, the uncertainty of Dave's course and the intensity of the treatment convinced me that I could not adequately commit to a clinical schedule. I traded my weeks on the inpatient service with a chief resident in exchange for me making the intern schedule, a task that I could accomplish remotely and at odd hours. You may have research or other educational/administrative responsibilities that you need to hand off. Make a plan for those, too.

Implement a communication strategy with your leadership team

Regular communication with my leadership team helped keep the program running. I didn't have an exact strategy at the beginning, with the flurry of activity and uncertainty as Dave's diagnosis and treatment plans unfolded. Once the transition into crisis was over, we developed a process that worked for us. Essentially, my program coordinator (PC) became my right-hand person. We met every Monday morning for an hour and reviewed the week's calendar, noting when I would be at work and when I anticipated being completely unavailable (i.e., the day of the transplant). My PC briefed me on need-to-know items, and we planned how to accomplish time-sensitive tasks. We decided what others could do and what I needed to do. This meeting set the stage for the week, allowing everyone to know what to expect. Predictability was very helpful to the leadership group and especially the residents. Of note, a trusted colleague suggested this strategy, underscoring the importance of leaning on others for advice during crises.

Choose a communication strategy for the whole program
Choices include a regular email to a specified group, routine virtual forums, or a blog, among others. Because our intention was to communicate with a wider audience beyond the residents, the blog made sense for us. It also allowed us flexibility to update it at our convenience. Pretty quickly, the online blog served as a place to give information, a source of connection, and a means to appreciate the many people who were supporting us. Over the course of David's illness, we received tremendous positive feedback for our blog.

Flashing forward to the COVID-19 pandemic, I drew upon these same communication strategies and principles to connect with our residents via nightly emails—content that provided information, funny anecdotes, random pop culture, and always ended with Three Good Things (Greater Good in Action, 2023). The principles of leadership through personal connection that I learned during David's illness directly translated to shepherding our residents through the early uncertainty and isolation of the COVID-19 pandemic.

Whatever communication strategy you choose, realize that transparency empowers others
Our transparency gave the residents agency by giving them the chance to help our family. This ranged from organizing a bone marrow registry together with a national organization, to signing up for a meal train (which we accepted), to volunteering to drive the kids to soccer practices (which we gracefully declined). Some residents sent notes, texts, or emails, and others made it a point to stop in the office to say hello whenever I was in. The residents' support was personally helpful. Having a group of 160 people behind you is very powerful. Because they were doctors, they understood; they could relate to someone who had a sick family member. We made it a point to mention frequently how important they were to us in our blog.

> "When residents see us living our lives out loud, processing terrifying and sad experiences, taking time away to be with sick loved ones, we make the hidden curriculum visible and actively challenge it."

In normal circumstances, it can be hard for residents to see their PD as a real person; we do not always show the residents the messy details of our lives. Through our crisis, we invited the residents into our most difficult moments. They were able to really see us. On one of my days at work, a junior resident came in to meet with me. As we talked, I received a message from Dave saying that his treatment plan had changed unexpectedly (and for the worse) based on results that had just returned. I started to cry, and she comforted me. The hidden curriculum in medicine says we must always be perfect and strong. When residents see us living our lives out loud, processing terrifying and sad experiences, taking time away to be with sick loved ones, we make the hidden curriculum visible, actively challenge it, and start relegating it to the past.

> **Communication Considerations**
>
> - How will you maintain communication with your leadership team?
> - How will you communicate with your residents?
> - How much personal information will you share?

Recognize that writing can bring personal benefit

I encourage anyone going through a crisis to incorporate a consistent writing practice into their daily routine. The blog began as a means of communication but became (perhaps selfishly) a way to process the overwhelming nature of our situation. A nurse friend of mine noticed that my blog entries became less clinical and more personal over time. I had not journaled regularly before this, certainly nothing intentional. While I love to read narrative medicine pieces ("A Piece of My Mind" in *JAMA* or "On Being a Doctor" in *Annals of Internal Medicine*), I was not a champion of reflective writing. Now I can see the therapeutic value in it, and the literature supports this observation: reflective writing is associated with improvements in health (Burton & King, 2008; Francis & Pennebaker, 1992). I closed out most days writing the blog, and when I finished, I felt prepared for the next day. I looked forward to writing each night and slept better once the day's entry was written. The responsive nature of the blog made the experience of writing it better, but I am certain that even writing it down on paper and not sharing it with anyone would still have been beneficial to me.

Know that staying connected to work can be a source of stability in times of personal crisis

I know that staying connected to work will resonate with some people in a similar situation, but it may not resonate with others. Also, there are other personal crises in which staying engaged in work simply may not make sense. For me, after the initial shock subsided, I realized that having some work to do was helpful for me at times. I also wanted residents to see that work can sometimes be a source of stability and joy during times of personal challenge.

> **Personal Considerations**
>
> - What does your family need?
> - Is work a source of stability or stress or both and what does that mean for staying connected to it?
> - How will you work through your own emotions (e.g., writing/journaling)?

Plan your re-entry to work

In the post-crisis phase, you will need to plan your "re-entry," which could vary from abrupt (should your crisis have a sharp dissipation) or gradual. When David returned to work himself, some seven months after diagnosis, that provided a natural boundary for my more complete return as well. Our first team meeting focused on thanking our team and collectively outlining the remaining tasks/schedule for the year. Through individual meetings with each APD, we added more detail to the transition (e.g., informing me of any need-to-know information and being transparent about what responsibilities I would resume).

Summary

Notably, one cannot stay in "crisis" mode indefinitely. The time from diagnosis to returning home was approximately nine months, with ebbs and flows of acuity and emotion. During the prolonged time of our family illness, both consistent physical presence as well as consistent virtual presence was helpful in maintaining a sense of stability for our residents as well as for me as I tried to balance the many roles of wife, parent, colleague, and program director. While fully "living one's life out loud" in terms of a frank and open blog is not for everyone, it was extremely valuable for sharing information. The blog echoed the principles of honesty, transparency, and stability that are familiar to us as key factors of success in our educational programs. There are other ways to model these same principles if you are reluctant to share as much as we did. While I did not know it at the time, my experience with the blog and the explicit core principles were invaluable to me (as they were to many of you) during the early part of the COVID-19 pandemic.

Living and leading through this crisis changed me as a leader. I am more willing to share the real "me" than I was in the past. I understand deeply the value of accepting the support offered by others in times of personal crisis. I was amazed and humbled by the care and empathy that residents displayed for us throughout our ordeal. And if you ever wonder about the impact that you are making as a PD, remember that we lived with our former PD during the transplant. The bond that develops between PDs and residents is strong and durable and has the capacity for enormous caring.

Table 2. Summary approach to personal crisis	
Pre-Crisis	• Cultivate trust, shared mental models, and deep organizational knowledge in your leadership team

Crisis	• Remember your own/your program's core values
	• Plan the disclosure to your residents
	• Outline the decisions that need to be made
	   - Do you need a LOA?
	   - Who can take some of your work responsibilities?
	   - What does your family need?
	   - Can you do clinical work during this crisis?
	• Plan your communication strategy
	• Find ways to take care of yourself
	• Allow others to support you

Post-Crisis	• Plan your re-entry to work • Show gratitude for the support that you received • Consider lessons learned that could be applied in the future

Citations

Burton, C. M., & King, L. A. (2008). Effects of (Very) Brief Writing on Health: The Two-Minute Miracle. *British Journal of Health Psychology, 13*(1), 9-14. https://doi.org/https://doi.org/10.1348/135910707X250910

Francis, M. E., & Pennebaker, J. W. (1992). Putting Stress into Words: The Impact of Writing on Physiological, Absentee, and Self-Reported Emotional Well-Being Measures. *American Journal of Health Promotion, 6*(4), 280-287. https://doi.org/10.4278/0890-1171-6.4.280

Greater Good in Action. (2023). *Three Good Things: A Way to Tune into the Positive Events in Your Life*. University of California, Berkeley. Retrieved May 18, 2023 from https://ggia.berkeley.edu/practice/three-good-things

Manning, K. (2022). *In Times of Crisis, Managers Must Develop a New Skill: Grief Leadership*. Fast Company. Retrieved May 31, 2023 from https://www.fastcompany.com/90719917/in-times-of-crisis-managers-must-develop-a-new-skill-grief-leadership

CHAPTER 10

Taking Care of Yourself During a Crisis

Mariah Quinn, MD, MPH

Mary Westergaard, MD

Art Walaszek, MD

University of Wisconsin School of Medicine and Public Health

In this chapter, the authors address the emotional toll of being the program director during a crisis. They offer suggestions for how to personally prepare for a crisis and how to find the resilience you need to get through the crisis. Preparation, self-awareness, and connection are essential to taking care of yourself during a crisis.

Introduction

A key responsibility of academic medical center leaders is to support healthcare professionals. Strong leaders care about their colleagues and appreciate that such support allows healthcare professionals to care for patients more effectively. Shanafelt and colleagues argue that "it is critical that leaders understand the sources of concern, assure healthcare professionals that their concerns are recognized, and work to develop approaches that mitigate concerns to the extent that they are able" (T. Shanafelt et al., 2020). This is especially important during a crisis.

Program directors (PDs) are charged with the care and support of residents and fellows. During times of crisis, this can be especially stressful for PDs, who may experience burnout. Lack of support from leadership is a factor for PDs who consider resigning. In a high-functioning organization, leaders such as chairs, vice chairs for education, deans, and hospital leaders should offer support when a PD is struggling. What happens if PDs get inadequate support? The pandemic has sharpened the focus on this question as reports surface of PDs struggling to protect their residents without any such protection for themselves (Fletcher et al.).

In this chapter, we suggest how PDs can find support and take care of themselves during times of crisis. We present three stories to illustrate support before, during, and after crises. The names we use and situations we describe do not represent actual people or events.

Story#1: The Handoff

Since 2009, the median tenure of an internal medicine program director has ranged from four to six years (O'Connor et al., 2019). Walking to her office for one last meeting to discuss the handoff, I wondered how my predecessor had happily served in the role for nearly 20 years. As the newly appointed residency PD, I knew there would be challenges, but I honestly could not imagine a better career. This is what I had always wanted, and I felt prepared and confident—in my ideas and innovations, my ability to connect with the residents, and my ability to work very, very hard at the things that matter to me. My administrative skillset was pretty good, too, and I didn't mind the issues that others perceived as major headaches. Every job has its own set of challenges and rewards, after all.

As I walked into her tidy office, Dr. Jones redirected me from the desk to a more comfortable corner table, a move that told me this was going to be a different type of handoff conversation. She opened by saying that it's important to talk about PD burnout. She wanted to share her lived experience of how a PD can be thriving on the outside and suffering on the inside. Most notably, she said, it was important to frame things for me in case I encountered similar struggles.

Her first rough patch as PD came five years in, after the call schedule had changed. It was certainly the better call schedule for the program, but it unavoidably put the senior residents at a disadvantage during the transition. Rejecting well-intentioned mitigation tactics, and spurred on by a charismatic peer, a cohort of residents became increasingly and publicly disgruntled about multiple aspects of the training program. A tsunami of negativity ensued: residents were unhappy and gossiping, each of the classes had myriad complaints, and the all-important ACGME resident survey took a nosedive. The aftermath was humiliating. Dr. Jones described her shame at the program's dissection in front of the Graduate Medical Education Committee, and all the extra work that came with a special site visit. She described how personal it all felt, the loneliness of having to pretend she was fine so the program could be fine, too. She won a prestigious national teaching award that year, but there was no joy in receiving it, just the shame at feeling like a fraud.

Thankfully, Dr. Jones survived with the help of the department chair. Over time, she successfully turned around the surveys and overall climate. Then, about five years later, a similar period of unrest emerged, with similar themes. "Bottom line," she said, "is that changes are tumultuous, and you should think about how to prepare for the inevitable periods of unrest and unpopularity coming your way." She said that being a good steward of the program might entail sacrificing one's ego a bit, but that strong mentorship and commitment to self-care would see me through. As I left her office, I found myself confident in the mentorship piece but unsure about "self-care." In all honesty, I did not achieve all that I had (including being selected for PD) by prioritizing self-care.

Advice from the Literature and Practical Wisdom

The internal work of resilience for PDs

New PDs know they will be held accountable for myriad policies and procedures stemming from both external and internal graduate medical education regulations. However, deliberately creating and maintaining a system for the PD's self-care is not an ACGME requirement beyond well-being for faculty members in general. It is also not a topic that residency leaders typically prioritize with so many competing demands. Establishing a system for self-care early on constitutes essential preventive care for individuals leading residency programs and should be approached deliberately.

Crises are the rule, not the exception

The first step in preparing to lead through crises is expecting that crises will occur. New PDs may expect their new role to consist largely of what is in their job description, but when catastrophe strikes, the job must pivot accordingly. At times, this is at the expense of the routine PD tasks (which of course still need to be done). Rather than lament the substantial new workload associated with managing crises, effective PDs will shift their mindset to recognize that crisis management is the job. They activate their supports at home and at work, and delegate tasks decisively and without guilt to be fully present for the most important work.

During crises, high emotion is to be expected, and even desired. Depending on the scenario, a PD may feel sadness, grief, or outrage at injustice. Other distressing emotions may include feeling overwhelmed ("I don't have time for this!"), fear ("I'm going to lose my job over this"), guilt ("I should have seen this coming, it's all my fault"), or defensiveness ("I didn't create this problem"). Imposter syndrome ("I'm not a good enough leader for this job") can also affect PDs. While understandable, such ruminations can detract from effective leadership. Of course, each of us must decide which emotions are helpful and which are not. Consider seeking the help of a therapist if negative emotions persist.

Building emotional awareness
Emotional awareness is a tool that is as important as it is underappreciated. Knowing whether a particular emotion is serving or hindering you (as recommended above) requires that you have awareness of your emotions in the first place. Building this awareness takes time and practice. New PDs are already in a state of transition, and this is a perfect opportunity to begin new practices to support emotional awareness. Journaling and mindfulness practice are two valuable tools that can be used to gain insight into one's thoughts and emotions. There is no need to sugarcoat or try to change what is unfolding in one's brain, but building the skill of awareness will be invaluable when crises strike. PDs with emotional insight will know when their thoughts and emotions are not serving their goals. Over time, they will learn to shift their attention away from less productive thoughts and toward thoughts that spur needed action.

By developing emotional awareness, PDs may be better prepared to protect their core identity from being disturbed by short-lived changes in their thinking and emotions. The ability to see circumstances, thoughts, and emotions as transient and separate from one's sense of self is a tenet of mindfulness practice. It can play a vital role for self-preservation during devastating events.

Many PDs have very high expectations for themselves and low self-compassion, which can make it more difficult to let go of self-defeating responses to crises. Seeing these responses as an understandable part of the human condition and maintaining a stance of gentleness toward themselves rather than self-judgment allows a PD with higher self-compassion to move into a state of curiosity and growth (Lanaj et al.; T. D. Shanafelt et al., 2020).

Self-care habits

Becoming a new PD is a major transition that lends itself to the establishment of new habits, which may or may not be associated with the position. Given that crises are the rule, and strong emotion is to be expected, it is wise to leverage this transition to build new routines, which foster resilience. Adequate sleep is critical for performance and emotional regulation; sleep impairment is associated with burnout (Trockel et al., 2020). Many physicians cite exercise as vital to their sense of well-being. Adopting an exercise routine is a wise investment for overall well-being. For example, a daily walk outside gives the added benefit of natural light and surroundings to expand one's horizons when work is all-consuming. Ultimately, self-care habits are highly individual. It is vital to identify, implement, and prioritize self-care activities. PDs should spend time to delineate rejuvenating, non-work activities and commit to incorporating them into their lifestyles. Likewise, non-work priorities should be faithfully incorporated into one's schedule, so they don't get dropped when work responsibilities surge.

Strengthen your network

In addition to developing self-care skills, it is helpful for a PD to preserve existing relationships and cultivate new relationships with other trusted PDs at their (or other) institution(s), as well as other leaders. This network of trusted supporters and advisers will lift you up when challenges inevitably arise.

As we move into new phases of life, we tend to focus on the people in front of us, sometimes to the detriment of longstanding friendships. Old friends can be invaluable anchors in tumultuous times. We view some of our own co-residents almost as siblings because of the intensity of our time together. Staying connected can help you remember your values and the hard lessons you have already learned. Their enduring regard and proven belief in you can be sustaining when you feel judged by each action and decision in the highly visible role as PD. Similarly, explicitly nurture your family relationships. They, too, have known you in better and worse times and can be a source of refuge when you need it.

Leaders need a deep network of peers. National organizations such as the Association of Program Directors in Surgery, the American Association of Directors of Psychiatric Residency Training, and the Association of Program Directors in Internal Medicine offer resources, listservs, and annual meetings for networking (and peer support!). Peer leaders from outside your organization provide perspective and fresh insight when you are facing difficult problems. The toolkits and development resources are also helpful, so participating in national organizations is essential. Cultivate relationships with other leaders at your institution as well. They understand the local politics and microculture, adding valuable and accessible sources of support and advice. It has been said that the quality of your day is directly proportional to the number of people you greet on the way to your office, so cast your institutional net wide.

Remember that a strong network may very well include having a therapist. We frequently encourage our trainees to seek mental health care; sometimes we need to take that advice ourselves.

Attend to personal mental health

Burnout, depression, and anxiety are common among PDs. Preventing or reducing these directly through the behaviors described is of critical importance. However, formal counseling and therapy can and should be normalized and utilized. When PDs access mental health services and speak about the benefits of doing so, they help to reduce stigma for others who will benefit from seeking mental health services as well (Brower, 2021).

Build skills in change management

Since change necessitates adaptation, it often is accompanied by stress for individuals and groups. Learning skills in change management not only helps a PD anticipate the likely phases of a group's response to change, but also provides a framework of skills to navigate these more successfully (Anderson, 2022; Kotter, 1996).

> **Story #2: Building a Resilient Team**
>
> *As I assumed the PD role, I leveraged my generally proactive approach to consider what actions might help me remain resilient. Especially after my conversation with Dr. Jones, I wanted to continue being an effective leader and steward of my team. I sought wisdom from respected colleagues. I specifically sought mentorship from PDs who had been in the role for at least five years, including Dr. Azaki, who had been a PD for 10 years. I knew her to be capable, positive, thoughtful, and kind. She agreed to go for a walk to answer new questions I had after considering Dr. Jones' advice. Specifically, I noted that crises came up from time to time; I wondered what steps she took when facing a crisis. She shared that she was recruited to our institution in the*

wake of a very difficult crisis in her prior role as an Associate PD (APD) at another institution. A resident had developed acute behavioral changes, which were reported by a faculty member to another APD when the PD was away. A very difficult series of conversations followed, and decisions had to be made quickly. Dr. Azaki shared that the APDs worried the PD did not appreciate their grave concerns; that the PD was not adequately engaged. Upon returning, the PD did become involved, but the feelings of disconnectedness persisted. Several parallel narratives emerged, each person with their own version of the story. The sharing of the many relational, communication, and coordination burdens was disjointed. Each team member was impacted; each needed help, reassurance, support, and appreciation. Each felt isolated with fear and worry. Each questioned whether what others had done was correct, or enough. There was even an air of competition as resentments grew: who had done what, when, and for whom; who had spent the most hours on the circumstance?

As the situation came to a difficult resolution and became part of memory, so too did each team member's isolating and fragmented experience. Instead of the crisis uniting and strengthening their team, it had further opened long-standing wounds. Dr. Azaki felt that changes in the dynamics of the team, facilitated by the PD, could have gone a long way toward helping the team work productively together and support one another.

When Dr. Azaki had the chance to apply for her current role, she saw it as an opportunity to build a team that could work together effectively, even when significant challenges arose. Prior to starting as PD, Dr. Azaki had taken a leadership course that focused on building and maintaining an effective team. Indeed, Dr. Azaki's team of APDs, program coordinator, and chief residents became widely seen as a uniquely high-functioning team. They were academically productive in educational scholarship and managed issues in their program while advocating for their own residents and other trainees. They also seemed to genuinely like one another. What she was doing as a PD was working.

Advice from the Literature and Practical Wisdom
Individuals to team: Laying the foundation

When a new PD starts, it is critical to establish positive relationships with APDs, the program coordinator, and any other program staff. The leadership behaviors of the PD can be expected to significantly impact the well-being and performance of team members. (T. D. Shanafelt et al., 2020). To establish these relationships, it is helpful to have regular, brief (generally 15-20 minutes) one-on-one meetings with the APDs, in addition to group meetings. These meetings initially should be focused on getting to know the APDs as people, as well as to understand what they are passionate about and working on. Once this knowledge is established, these meetings can focus on what is working well, what isn't working well, anything else the PD should know about, and how the PD can help. The APDs may let the PD know what she should be doing more, less, or stop doing. These connections should not only pave the way for APD success but also increase psychological safety. Finally, the PD can model that discussing self-care and personal well-being is expected and necessary.

Group meetings should be organized to not only keep everyone informed about important changes at the institution or at the ACGME, but to encourage conversation and dialogue as well as respect for the time and efforts of each member of the team. Feedback, appreciation, and recognition should be distributed liberally and regularly. Discussing and negotiating how to best communicate during and between meetings should be revisited as a regular topic, especially if challenges emerge.

Consider having periodic retreats with your leadership team. Retreats can be used to develop the glacial resources described in Chapter 1, such as trust and shared mental models. You can also use this time to establish program priorities and corresponding goals. APDs often want clarity about their specific roles. Retreats are a good time to realign APD resources to the program's strategic priorities.

Managing the calendar
Speaking of meetings: PDs convene many meetings and are asked to participate in many meetings. Scheduling these meetings (and responding to others' requests for a list of your availability) can become a very time-consuming task, so we recommend delegating this task to an administrative assistant, program coordinator, or other staff member. You retain control over your calendar by deciding which meetings you want to attend before forwarding requests to your administrative assistant. Also, indicate the length of meetings that you initiate and the required attendees.

Even in the absence of a crisis, the daily schedule of a PD can be very demanding. It can threaten to cut into well-established personal priorities and self-care habits. Another wise investment with wide-ranging benefits for PDs is committing to elevating time management skills. While administrative skills are recognized as important for PDs, they are not often taught in a systematic way. Shifting from keeping to-do lists to calendaring is an effective time management method with substantial efficiencies. Calendaring generally involves setting aside a regularly recurring time (typically weekly) to collate all to-do list activities and add them to one's calendar, with a firm commitment to doing exactly what is planned during each time slot (Allen, 2015; Becker, 2023). Make sure to include time on your calendar to work on big projects too, so that you spend time on important, but not urgent, tasks. It is easy for a PD to constantly put out fires. Blocking time for other work is essential to success and fulfillment (Covey, 1989).

It is wise to prioritize scheduling both self-care and personal responsibilities. (As flight attendants wisely advise, put your own oxygen mask on first!) Scheduling sleep directly on the calendar can be an effective nudge and promote optimal functioning. Regularly calendaring will ensure the PD is prioritizing their available time rather than constantly reacting to others' agendas. Of course, during crisis, there will often be unexpected demands on a PD's time, but this, too, can be managed with pre-planned "overflow" time. It is important to remain in control of the calendar; to thoughtfully choose how to spend one's time. Calendaring is a wise early-career investment that will mature over time.

The duality of PD as peer and leader
A PD is both peer and leader to the APDs, and PDs must be thoughtful about navigating this duality, forming authentic relationships while being aware of the force of hierarchy. They must pay attention to the impact their words and actions have on the team. Their influence is outsized, and what they say and do have an effect that can reach beyond their intention. When there is a misstep or mistake, address it openly with the team, take accountability, and model appropriate vulnerability—all of which sets the stage for psychological safety. The ability of leaders to acknowledge their own vulnerability, missteps, uncertainty—and to share sincere acknowledgment of the efforts of other team members—requires emotional awareness and self-regulation.

Story #3: A Tragedy in the Program

It was 3:00 AM, and my department chair was calling. Emma, the wife of one of our residents, John, was in the emergency department following a motor vehicle accident and was not expected to survive. Emma and John were an outgoing couple well known to many residents, faculty, and staff across the hospital. They had regularly attended our department's social events, and some of their closest friends were residents in our program.

I rushed to the ED and found it silent. Attempts to resuscitate Emma had ended minutes earlier. John sat outside the room, head in hands, surrounded by many of his fellow residents. I felt lightheaded, and my mouth dried out as I fumbled condolences. I nodded acknowledgment of the other residents there and stepped away for a few minutes to update the chair and our APDs. When I returned, John and the other residents had moved into a family room just outside the ED. A chaplain joined them. I awkwardly stood in a corner of the room, trying not to cry, mentally drafting the email I would send to our department, feeling nauseous about the painful conversations that would come next. After an hour or so, I excused myself and returned home for a brief, fitful sleep.

Over the next week, I found it painful and dissonant trying to lead a residency program through a traumatic event while also grieving myself. How could I be visible and available to residents, communicate with them effectively, refer them to available resources, and address the administrative details of academic medicine while I was still feeling shocked at the sudden loss of a bright young woman in her twenties and tearing up whenever I called John to check in on him? I was disappointed in myself for being selfish and not stoic enough. I had such great mentors—Dr. Jones, Dr. Azaki, my chair, many others—and I was falling short and failing my residents. I felt guilty. What right did I have to grieve when John had just lost his wife and our residents had just lost their friend?

It was in this frame of mind that I went to Emma's memorial service. It seemed that the entire medical center was there, including all the residents in our program and many of our faculty. Many friends and family members described their sadness, shared their memories of Emma, even offered hope. Rows and rows of dark suits and black dresses were pressed together, yet grieving in their own ways.

Afterward, I approached Emma's parents and sisters, John by their side. Before I could say anything, he enveloped me in a hug and said, "Thank you for being there for me." It was okay to cry, and I did.

Advice from the Literature and Practical Wisdom

Loss, grief, and the program director

We suspect there are many right ways to lead residents through a crisis. A crisis may be a loss—the loss of a fellow human being or the loss of how things used to be. Grief is the normal human reaction to loss. Everyone facing the crisis, including the PD, will experience grief, which can show up as sadness, anger, withdrawing from friends and family, avoiding painful emotions or reminders, and many other ways. Accepting the universality of grief won't make dealing with a crisis any easier, but it will help PDs navigate in a more humane and authentic manner.

Leaders, including PDs, play a critical role in helping their communities recover following tragedies: "As shock and horror turn to sorrow and mourning, leaders are responsible for identifying the timing of when a community is ready for the next step forward and how best to speak the language of each community to help individuals, families, and care providers" (Center for the Study of Traumatic Stress).

In the immediate aftermath of a tragedy like Emma's death, a PD should be visible and should provide accurate and timely information (to the extent allowable), using multiple means of communication (e.g., phone trees, email, group chats) (Center for the Study of Traumatic Stress). PDs should be aware of and share resources, such as the local employee assistance program, Peer Support program, and the ACGME's "After a Suicide Toolkit" (Dyrbye et al., 2016).

While the story above stopped at the PD attending the memorial service (an important step in and of itself), the recovery may continue for weeks, months, or longer. During recovery, the PD should work with departmental and institutional leadership to "establish a climate of healing and community support" (Center for the Study of Traumatic Stress). When the time is right, the PD can lead the residents and faculty in "respectful remembering and recovery efforts" (Center for the Study of Traumatic Stress). It is essential to remember that "recovery takes time, is not linear," and varies quite a bit from person to person (Center for the Study of Traumatic Stress). The PD also may be grieving and will need to engage in their own recovery.

Summary

What a program director actually does is often very different from their job description and from what the ACGME requirements state. This is especially true of the emotional and relational work necessary to support residents and guide residency and fellowship programs through crises. While being a PD is among the most professionally and personally rewarding experiences in academic medicine, frequent crises could result in burnout and high turnover.

We propose that PDs prepare for and respond to crises by adopting three sets of practices. First, PDs should establish a system of self-care that includes good sleep, exercise, healthy relationships, and setting aside time for personal activities. Once a PD accepts that managing crises is one of the most important parts of her job, she can build emotional awareness: naming emotions and moving away from unproductive thoughts to effective actions. Second, PDs must manage a team of colleagues, including offering necessary support and mentoring, acknowledging mistakes, modeling vulnerability, and recognizing the efforts of the members of the team. Managing a calendar, with administrative support, is essential for having the time necessary for both self-care and the care of the rest of the team. Third, PDs may have to lead in the midst and aftermath of a devastating loss, while others are grieving and they themselves are grieving, too. While PDs can take steps to prepare before such a crisis and to lead during the crisis, it is essential to acknowledge the many forms of grief and to participate in community rituals to help address grief.

PDs can serve as models of effective leadership during crises, caring both for themselves and those around them.

Table 1. Summary approach to taking care of yourself during a crisis	
Pre-Crisis	Build a strong team
	Strengthen your network of outside support
	Implement a plan for calendar/workload management
	Develop and practice self-care habits (sleep, exercise, relationships)
	Develop personal resilience and emotional awareness
	Attend to personal mental health
	Build skills in change management
Crisis	Hone and implement change management skills
	Call on your personal resilience
	Use emotional awareness skills
	Continue to use calendar/workload management plan
	Maintain self-care habits
	Attend to personal mental health
	Support and attend to your team
	Engage your network of supportive peers
Post-Crisis	Attend to personal recovery and mental health
	Facilitate the team's recovery
	Reflect on the crisis as a team
	Lead a discussion of what your team learned

Citations

Allen, D. D. (2015). Getting Things Done: The Art of Stress-Free Productivity (Revised edition. ed.). Penguin Books.

Anderson, E. (2022). Change Is Hard. Here's How to Make It Less Painful. *Harvard Business Review*. https://hbr.org/2022/04/change-is-hard-heres-how-to-make-it-less-painful

Becker, C. (2023). Timeboxing – why you should use it? Firmbee. Retrieved May 15, 2023 from https://firmbee.com/timeboxing-why-you-should-use-it#firstparagraph

Brower, K. J. (2021). Professional Stigma of Mental Health Issues: Physicians Are Both the Cause and Solution. *Acad Med, 96*(5), 635-640. https://doi.org/10.1097/acm.0000000000003998

Center for the Study of Traumatic Stress. (2021). Grief Leadership: Leadership in the Wake of Tragedy. https://www.cstsonline.org/assets/media/documents/CSTS_FS_Grief_Leadership_in_theWake_of_Tragedy.pdf

Covey, S. R. (1989). The Seven Habits of Highly Effective People: Restoring the Character Ethic. Simon and Schuster. http://catdir.loc.gov/catdir/enhancements/fy0705/89030464-s.html

Dyrbye, L., Konopasek, L., & Moutier, C. V., for the American Foundation for Suicide Prevention (2017). *After a Suicide: A Toolkit for Physician Residency/Fellowship Programs*. American Foundation for Suicide Prevention. https://www.acgme.org/globalassets/pdfs/13287_afsp_after_suicide_clinician_toolkit_final_2.pdf

Fletcher, K. E., Finn, K. M., Kiselewski, M., Simmons, R., Zaas, A., & Zetkulic, M. (2022). The Trauma of the COVID-19 Pandemic: Impact on Residency Program Directors. Fall Association of Program Directors in Internal Medicine Meeting.

Kotter, J. P. (1996). Leading Change. Harvard Business School Press.

Lanaj, K., Foulk, T. A., & Jennings, R. E. (2023). Improving the Lives of Leaders: The Beneficial Effects of Positive Leader Self-Reflection. *Journal of Management, 48*(8), 2595-2628. https://doi.org/10.1177/01492063221110205

O'Connor, A. B., Halvorsen, A. J., Cmar, J. M., Finn, K. M., Fletcher, K. E., Kearns, L., McDonald, F. S., Swenson, S. L., Wahi-Gururaj, S., West, C. P., & Willett, L. L. (2019). Internal Medicine Residency Program Director Burnout and Program Director Turnover: Results of a National Survey. *Am J Med, 132*(2), 252-261. https://doi.org/10.1016/j.amjmed.2018.10.020

Shanafelt, T., Ripp, J., & Trockel, M. (2020). Understanding and Addressing Sources of Anxiety among Health Care Professionals during the COVID-19 Pandemic. *Jama, 323*(21), 2133-2134. https://doi.org/10.1001/jama.2020.5893

Shanafelt, T. D., Makowski, M. S., Wang, H., Bohman, B., Leonard, M., Harrington, R. A., Minor, L., & Trockel, M. (2020). Association of Burnout, Professional Fulfillment, and Self-Care Practices of Physician Leaders With Their Independently Rated Leadership Effectiveness. *JAMA Netw Open, 3*(6), e207961. https://doi.org/10.1001/jamanetworkopen.2020.7961

Trockel, M. T., Menon, N. K., Rowe, S. G., Stewart, M. T., Smith, R., Lu, M., Kim, P. K., Quinn, M. A., Lawrence, E., Marchalik, D., Farley, H., Normand, P., Felder, M., Dudley, J. C., & Shanafelt, T. D. (2020). Assessment of Physician Sleep and Wellness, Burnout, and Clinically Significant Medical Errors. *JAMA Netw Open, 3*(12), e2028111. https://doi.org/10.1001/jamanetworkopen.2020.28111

CHAPTER 11

Recovering from a Leadership Misstep

David L. Hamel, Jr., MD, FACP

Aurora Health Care

This chapter outlines principles to apply after a leadership mistake and provides perspective on identifying and preventing future mistakes. The author suggests that making a leadership mistake can be a golden opportunity for leaders to build trust, psychological safety, shared mental models, and other resource stocks to prepare for the next crisis.

Introduction

Whether you are a new program director (PD) or a seasoned one, chances are you've made your share of mistakes. "To err is human" has been an oft-repeated phrase in our profession since the Institute of Medicine, in their 1999 report, borrowed the line from the poet Alexander Pope. Our goal as leaders is not to strive for unerring perfection, but to learn how to respond to our failures in a way that builds our team's culture, resource stocks, and ability to respond to change. In fact, human development and psychology researchers have shown us that how you respond to—or, in their words, repair—a mistake is more important to a relationship than whether you made the mistake in the first place (Morton, 2016). Recovering well after a leadership misstep may lead to a better relationship and reputation than "mistake-free" leadership.

Story: The Ill-Considered Policy Change

In March of 2021, one year into the COVID-19 pandemic, my chief residents and I were brainstorming how to make our virtual meetings and conferences more engaging. Our daily virtual noon conferences brought together 25 residents, but questions posed to the group were often followed by complete silence, until—awkwardly—speakers would answer their own questions. We suspected many residents were multitasking during conference time. One morning, after a brief meeting with the chief residents, I sent the following email to all program residents and faculty:

> *Subject: Zoom Video Policy Change*
>
> *Hi Team,*
>
> *We are looking for ways to boost engagement in noon conference. I notice that I am more engaged in meetings when my camera is on, and I hope you experience the same for your learning. Effective now, all program meetings and conferences will require participants to keep their video cameras on. This applies to both resident and faculty meetings. We will be evaluating the results of this policy change. You can expect a survey in two weeks asking for your feedback.*

The day before my next meeting with our faculty (in our small program, I also serve as department chair, overseeing faculty, residents, and clinical operations), I received a phone call from an associate program director (APD) saying that she thought the policy was right for the residents, but that the faculty should be exempt from needing to be on camera. I told her I believed strongly that we should lead by example, and if we thought it was good for the residents, it should apply to us as well. I felt self-assured I was doing the right thing. During the faculty meeting, most faculty members thought they should not be required to be on camera, citing several valid concerns. Our faculty meetings were after work hours, unlike noon conference. Many of our faculty had parenting responsibilities like school pickups and housework. The move to virtual meetings enhanced the "life" part of their work-life balance. They thought they could easily take in information and participate in discussion while driving or loading laundry. One faculty member asked if there were times I felt they weren't paying attention; whether someone missed an important announcement, or wasn't participating in the discussion. I honestly couldn't point to an example, and they were always quick to offer an opinion when called upon in meetings. Several discussed concerns that there may be gender and individual differences around the feelings of being on camera, which could make them anxious and unable to focus on the meeting. One faculty member, who thought our residents might be distracted during noon conferences by seeing themselves or others on camera, wasn't convinced it would lead to better learning and retention. Our transitional year PD pointed out that her residents also attend noon conference, and I had not consulted her. Thankfully, she was willing to support whatever I decided.

Ultimately, I decided to ditch the camera requirement for faculty meetings after work hours, but I asked the faculty to put their cameras on when attending noon conference. On the follow-up survey, residents mentioned that being on camera added stress and detracted from their learning. Because of the feedback from both faculty and residents, I never committed to accountability on this policy, and I'm still not sure whether camera on or off is the right call. Regardless, the decision was rash and uninformed. The feedback could easily have been elicited prior to implementing the policy. Because of this experience, I try to always seek feedback before acting on anything now. When I do, I nearly always get a perspective that I hadn't considered, and we make better decisions for our program. I learned this the hard way.

Advice from the Literature and Practical Wisdom
Use best practices when making leadership decisions

There's not one right way to lead, and no best way of making tough leadership decisions. Some decisions benefit from a democratic process, and sometimes leaders need to be authoritative when there is disagreement, discomfort, or urgency. However, there are some best practices that apply to most, if not all, leadership decisions. Having a shared mental model of values within your program can prevent leadership decision missteps. Consider drafting a set of core values or a mission statement at your annual program evaluation. With this buy-in from your people on the values that matter most, your future decisions will have an implicit justification: your program's values. Simon Sinek highlights this practice in his book *Start With Why* (Sinek, 2011). My decision to require video cameras to be on during virtual meetings in an effort to boost engagement may have been better received if I explained the "why" driving my decision. My chiefs and I discussed our desire to improve the educational value of noon conferences, but that message wasn't communicated clearly to residents and faculty. I host a monthly meeting with all residents called "Program Updates and Listening Session," where I explain the reasons for program or health system policy changes. In hindsight, waiting for one of those meetings would have been a much better way to announce this decision and provide context.

Conduct a "pre-mortem" on decisions

We all make leadership mistakes, and avoiding them entirely is impossible. However, you can employ Carol Dweck's concept of a growth mindset and/or use a "pre-mortem" analysis to avoid a future misstep (Dweck, 2012). In her book *Dare to Lead*, Brené Brown describes a growth mindset of "I'm not here to be right. I'm here to get it right."(Brown, 2018). Bringing that mantra into the daily work of leading your program will prevent some leadership mistakes, which often arise from failing to consider a perspective or failing to consider why you might be wrong. However, as in clinical medicine, don't let this humility paralyze you from acting on important problems (see "Don't confuse discontent with mistakes," below). A pre-mortem analysis can help you with this.

A pre-mortem analysis is an imaginary post-mortem that happens before the failure occurs in real life (Klein, 2007). Imagine ahead of time that your decision didn't work out, and then think about the ways your future self would explain the failure. This process can identify the main threats to the success of your leadership decisions and allow you to plan or account for them or to seek additional input. In my case, I could have started the pre-mortem by taking a moment to consider why requiring video cameras to be on during noon conference could be a terrible idea. Then, I might have considered the distraction factor and the discomfort I feel being on camera. Even if I wouldn't have guessed all the complaints that later arose, I would have had enough doubt to stop and wonder if this decision required a discussion and not an email.

Seek additional input

I did well to seek my chief residents' input on our Zoom video policy, but I didn't seek input from faculty or residents on this change. As laid out in Chapter 1, building trust requires the leader to gather and value the opinions of all constituents. Thankfully, we had enough psychological safety within our program that I eventually got the feedback I needed. If your problem is urgent, you may not have the time to gather feedback from everyone necessary. In that case, asking someone to play the dev-

Table 1. Preventing leadership mistakes

- Establish a strong team culture with shared mental models, trust, and psychological safety
- Start with a growth mindset—"I'm here to get it right, not be right."
- Know your own biases
- Seek input from all stakeholders and consult with trusted advisors before key decisions
- Do a "pre-mortem" analysis on decisions

il's advocate (another concept from Chapter 1) can serve to prevent some leadership missteps. Knowing yourself and your biases are invaluable tools in the devil's advocate process. Even better, have a group of trusted advisors with diverse perspectives. Their biases may be different from yours (and each other's) and can compensate for your own. Finally, having shared mental models can help during times when you fail to seek that input. Shared mental models develop over time within a group, and they should help you take the perspective of those affected by your leadership decisions. But they cannot replace the discussions that should occur before making a leadership decision. My faculty and I had a shared mental model of noon conference quality, but we didn't have the same guiding values and mental model with respect to our faculty meetings.

Table 2. After a leadership mistake
• Own the mistake
• Seek your supervisor's support
• Decide how (and with whom) to talk about it
• Share what you learned and commit to do better
• Normalize mistakes that others make

Own the mistake

When we make a mistake, the most important first step is to own it. If you mess up, fess up. This goes against our inclination to hide the error and hope no one finds out, which often feeds our impostor syndrome. Even if you could hide, taking ownership as a leader will be seen as strong leadership and will outweigh any reputational damage you'd take if the mistake is uncovered in any other way (Downer, 2018). In this process, be sure to let your supervisor know what happened, how you plan to address it, and be sure you have their support before sharing the situation with your program. This doesn't have to be a big deal. Don't plan a program-wide meeting for every miscommunication and failed policy. You can mention it in passing to your residents and faculty and shift to what you learned or what you're going to do differently. When I gave the results of our Zoom video policy feedback survey, I shared that there were concerns I should have considered. I told my faculty and residents that I had assumed we had shared mental models of the importance of quality noon conferences and how people felt about Zoom video, and I learned a valuable lesson about questioning similar assumptions in the future. Sharing what you learned models a growth mindset, and—coupled with a commitment to do better next time—is a powerful tool to build respect as a leader within your program.

Normalize making mistakes

Do this by congratulating teammates on trying something new, even if it didn't work out. A few years ago, our system pitched the idea of having a faculty member work within our urology clinic, providing primary care to men without a primary care physician. One of our early-career faculty took this on. After committing a year of Wednesday afternoons to the clinic with very low volumes and high no-show rates, we decided to give up. It wasn't at the core of our program's mission. I thanked him publicly for his commitment to a project that helped us build good will and a reputation of citizenship within our system. Not every pilot project will work out. At the same time, don't abandon every new project that is facing roadblocks. Commit to ensuring the success of those projects that drive at the heart of your program's mission and vision. Scott McNealy, former Stanford Business School professor and CEO of Sun Microsystems, once said, "I spend much less time and energy worrying about 'making the right decision' and much more time and energy ensuring that any decision I make turns out right" (Batista, 2013).

> *"When someone comes forward with a mistake of their own, share a time you made a similar mistake. This avoids creating a 'shame and blame' culture within your program—a culture of hiding mistakes—and shows that growth and improvement are possible."*

When someone comes forward with a mistake of their own, share a time you made a similar mistake. This avoids creating a "shame and blame" culture within your program—a culture of hiding mistakes—and shows that growth and improvement are possible ("If I did it once and *still* became a program leader, imagine what you can do!"). Psychological safety explains why Amy Edmonson's research has demonstrated that the hospital units with the best outcomes are often *also* the ones with the highest error reporting rates—those teams are willing to acknowledge mistakes (Edmondson, 1996). It's natural for a leader to worry that sharing their past mistakes could ruin the respect and reputation of competence they have with those they lead. Demonstrating vulnerability in this context doesn't ruin your reputation. It takes courage and gives your people a similar reputation to live up to. It shows them that despite (or because of) their mistake, they can still be or become competent and effective. Normalizing mistakes makes it more likely that someone on your team will share their own mistakes with you.

Don't confuse discontent with mistakes

Identifying a leadership mistake can be challenging. Negative emotions from your residents like discontent and anger could say more about the state of the person giving the feedback than the decision itself. So, don't assume every decision you make will be well-received.

> *"Leaders should expect many 'right' decisions to be received with skepticism or discontent."*

Many times, the tougher decisions are the right ones. Before labeling a leadership decision as a "mistake," be sure to reflect on disagreement and discontent. Decide if this represents information you failed to consider or information that makes a good case for a change in strategy. If so, you should accommodate this feedback or even alter your decision. However, in this case, your job is to ensure these feelings are heard and validated. Thank them for their perspective and ask for permission to share your point of view. Explain why, considering all perspectives, this is the best decision for your program. Don't expect to persuade them but thank them for allowing you the space to share your thoughts.

We all have left a feedback session knowing that constructive criticism is left unsaid. As a leader, don't assume the right feedback will necessarily make it to you. All leaders should have someone (or a group of "someones") they can trust to give honest, respectful, and objective feedback. Be sure to get their perspective before and after a decision is made and do it whether or not things are going well. Finally, watch for "the meeting after the meeting" as a sign that there's feedback you haven't heard or perspectives you haven't considered. If you know of side conversations, text chains, and phone calls that are going on, be sure to create a space for those opinions to be voiced or approach those people directly and make them feel heard and validated.

Summary

All leaders make mistakes. If you successfully navigate a mistake, you can actually build trust within your program and your leadership group. Use the pre-crisis time to build shared mental models and diversify the viewpoints represented in your leadership group to help prevent future mistakes. Realize that even good decisions can be met with discontent; that does not mean that you made a mistake.

Table 2. Summary approach to recovering from a leadership mistake	
Pre-Mistake	• Establish shared mental models • Build trust and psychological safety • Diversify the viewpoints in your group
During the Mistake	• Own the mistake • Commit to doing better • Obtain support of your supervisor
Post-Mistake	• Help others navigate their mistakes by normalizing the experience

Citations

Batista, E. (2013). Stop Worrying About Making the Right Decision. *Harvard Business Review*. Retrieved May 25, 2023 from https://hbr.org/2013/11/stop-worrying-about-making-the-right-decision

Brown, B. (2018). *Dare to Lead: Brave Work. Tough Conversations. Whole Hearts.* Vermillion.

Downer, K. (2018). Leadership Mistakes: 3 Things to Do When You Really Step In It. RapidStart Leadership. Retrieved May 25, 2023 from https://www.rapidstartleadership.com/leadership-mistakes/

Dweck, C. S. (2012). *Mindset: How You Can Fulfill Your Potential*. Robinson.

Edmondson, A. C. (1996). Learning from Mistakes is Easier Said Than Done: Group and Organizational Influences on the Detection and Correction of Human Error. *The Journal of Applied Behavioral Science, 32*(1), 5-28. https://doi.org/10.1177/0021886396321001

Klein, G. (2007). Performing a Project Premortem. *Harvard Business Review*. Retrieved May 25, 2023 from https://hbr.org/2007/09/performing-a-project-premortem

Morton, M. (2016). We Can Work it Out: The Importance of Rupture and Repair Processes in Infancy and Adult Life for Flourishing. *Health Care Analysis, 24*(2), 119-132. https://doi.org/10.1007/s10728-016-0319-1

Sinek, S. (2011). *Start with Why: How Great Leaders Inspire Everyone to Take Action*. Portfolio / Penguin.

CHAPTER 12

Resident/Chief Resident Essays about Crisis

WHAT I LEARNED ABOUT MYSELF AND MY TEAM IN MY FIRST CRISIS AS A RESIDENT

Rachel Goodman, MD

Tufts University School of Medicine

Dr. Goodman looks back on an experience from her second year of internal medicine residency at the Medical College of Wisconsin when she was one of the responders after a visitor was shot on the medical campus. She describes the chaos and unexpected stress of being on lockdown. She prioritized debriefing with her team, even as she was trying to process the event herself.

After a long July day admitting patients, I finally had a moment to breathe. It was the middle of a 28-hour shift—only my second as a team leader—and I sat in my team room excited to eat my dinner that was now cold. My co-resident and friend who was also working overnight joined me from her post in the ICU. We spent the next few minutes reflecting on cases we had seen, asking for advice, and eating pasta we had ordered for delivery to the hospital. The rest of the team sat beside us, finishing notes and winding down before leaving for the night. Pagers were alarming with questions about insulin dosing and antibiotic timing.

I hadn't yet finished my pasta when a voice on the overhead public-address system announced, "Medical emergency, code team needed." I dropped my fork, grabbed my stethoscope, and ran downstairs to my first code as a senior resident. My heart was racing and my gym shoes were squeaking as I ran across the freshly cleaned floors. The ICU resident ran beside me, along with my intern and medical student who followed closely behind. We made our way to the emergency department, questioning the location as we ran. Codes were not generally called in the emergency department. Something was different.

We arrived at the code to find police officers lining the entrance to the emergency department. The high-pitched sounds of their walkie-talkies were faint in comparison to the yelling coming from inside the room. The handful of hospital staff sitting outside the trauma bay looked alarmed. They were whispering to each other, though not very quietly. I heard mention of guns and a shooting. The words "activate the massive transfusion protocol" came from inside.

I stepped inside. The chaos and confusion I sensed outside the room paled in comparison to what I saw inside the trauma bay. Nurses were running and techs were yelling. There was a line of people doing chest compressions. It was not clear if there was a physician in the room, let alone anyone running the code.

As the ICU resident in charge of running codes, my co-resident quickly took over. I stood beside her, collecting information to try to better understand what was happening. I learned that there was a shooting on the hospital grounds, and this was the victim. Police came in and out of the room, periodically checking in and filling in details that I only somewhat heard. The intern and medical students were peering in from the doorframe. The next thing I remember is placing my hand on the patient's leg and being surprised that it was warm. At the next pulse check, there was a palpable pulse. Once he was stable, the emergency room team taking care of him coordinated the rest of his care. He was transferred to our main hospital—a level 1 trauma center—where the surgeons would likely immediately take him to the operating room.

When I left the emergency department, we still did not know the circumstances of the shooting, but no one had indicated that there was a shooter at large. I slowly wandered back through the empty hallways in silence—my heart still racing and my gym shoes still squeaking. The rest of my team had already gone upstairs; some had even left the hospital campus. As I walked toward the team room, I saw two nurses huddled together, comforting each other. I walked inside to find one intern and one medical student still there. Neither of them said anything, but I could tell from the look in their eyes that they were scared and confused. I was, too. So, we debriefed. I don't remember what I said, but I remember feeling that this was an opportunity to check in with my team. I quickly realized that it is hard to lead a debrief when you aren't exactly sure what happened or how you are feeling, but I kept going and we kept talking. Soon after our debrief, our attending and program director called to check in. We talked about what I knew and how I was doing. In hindsight, I think I was too stunned to have an emotional reaction. She offered to come into the hospital to debrief in person, which I said was not necessary. She then spoke to every team member and internal medicine resident at the hospital at the time, whether or not they were directly involved.

Just following our conversation, an overhead announcement was made that the hospital was on lockdown. Nurses were crying in the hallway. Call lights and bed alarms were still ringing. Still too stunned to have an emotional reaction, I focused on the reason I was at work that night: to take care of patients. I ran the list, reviewed orders, and did a deep dive on prior diagnoses and hospitalizations. I kept pausing to check in with my team, though I was unsure what to ask. The lockdown ended, and we eventually learned that the victim had walked up to the hospital entrance with a gun, threatening to shoot, and had himself been shot by the campus police.

Following the lockdown, the remaining intern and medical student decided to go home for the night. I remember feeling unsure if this was the safest option because the circumstances of the shooting still seemed unclear, but I also recognized that it was not my decision to make. I asked them both to text me once they were in their cars, which they did.

The rest of the night continued as any other, focused on problem-solving and admitting patients. I went home the next morning and slept for over twelve hours—the mental exhaustion finally catching up with me. I have always joked that I thrive in chaotic situations, but it is less thriving and more the ability to push aside the chaos and focus on the task at hand. I'm not sure that is the best response. While I did not check in with my own feelings, I somehow recognized the importance of checking in with my team and giving them the space to process. Looking back, I wish I would have recognized that as chaotic as this situation was for all of us, my intern and medical student were simultaneously navigating a new job in a new system. Yes, I am calm in chaotic situations, but my ability to compartmentalize in this situation was likely aided by a familiarity with the system in which I was working.

Having now had years to reflect on the situation, here is what I have learned:

1. Take a breath.
2. Recognize that people respond to crisis differently, and that other aspects of their lives and situations likely impact these responses.
3. Leadership is more than standing at a podium and leading meetings. Behind the scenes is most important—the phone calls, the checking in, and the opportunities for reflection.

FINDING STRENGTH TOGETHER:
WEATHERING A NATURAL DISASTER WITH COLLEAGUES

Lawrence P.A. DeBellis, DO, MS

Medical University of South Carolina

In September 2022, Dr. DeBellis was a chief resident for his internal medicine residency program at the Naples Community Hospital in Naples, FL. He tells the story of planning for, working through, and regrouping after Hurricane Ian and its subsequent storm surge.

In September 2017, Hurricane Irma was a category 5 hurricane that swept across Florida, causing extensive damage to the Naples area. Our internal medicine residency was in its infancy at the time—in its second year—and our hurricane policy adopted at the dawn of our program had not been revised. To protect our residents, the policy stated that only senior residents could opt in for hurricane coverage. We did not have a specific protocol to utilize residents, and most residents were sent home in times of emergency.

By Hurricane Ian in September 2022, our program had grown by leaps and bounds. We had a more robust internal medicine residency program with a full complement of residents, a transitional year program, and fellowship programs, but any of the senior residents who had gone through Hurricane Irma had graduated and moved on. When reports of the hurricane started with a planned landfall a few hours north of Naples, we began discussions on how to prepare for the storm, both as a hospital and as a residency program. It was decided that residents would opt in to provide coverage for our patients.

Wednesday early afternoon

As one of the chief residents, I participated in a meeting with the GME administration, and we learned from our designated institutional officer (DIO) and assistant DIO that the hospital wanted to send all residents home. The hospital couldn't provide lodging, childcare, or pet care for all of the physicians across the hospital and academic program. This decision by administration made us realize that even though the program had expanded, emergency coverage policies had not been adjusted to account for that growth. We felt a "re-introduction" to our GME program was in order, but that would have to wait. All residents were told that it was optional to stay at the hospital overnight Wednesday during the storm; however, it was expected that everyone show up for their shift the next day, regardless of circumstances. Because we had limited space in our call rooms, our program decided to focus on keeping only senior residents in-house.

I was tasked to find volunteers, in addition to seniors already in-house, to cover the critical care unit and the general medicine resident patients in the hospital. The seniors who were already on the wards and unit expected this, although without interns we needed additional volunteers. Many residents ignored my call. However, some pulled me aside and said, "If you need me, I will be there." While those residents didn't want to openly volunteer, they respected that I volunteered to stay overnight and work alongside them. We were able to house five residents for the medicine/surgery floors, two residents covering the ICU, and the pulmonology critical care fellow. One of the academic hospitalists stayed over. I also stayed to centralize GME communications and act as an additional attending in the event our other attending physicians on the schedule that week could not get back to the hospital. Our census at the time was too much for one attending.

Wednesday late afternoon

After arranging and scheduling volunteers, I had only a few hours to leave the hospital, stormproof my home, and ransack it for snacks to get me through the night. I quickly grabbed anything from home that I thought could be useful, including flashlights, batteries, cases of water, and nonperishable foods. I will admit, I was not as prepared with resources as I should have been because the original forecast put the storm two and a half hours north of us. I did not stop to purchase additional supplies because I wanted to get back to the hospital before they restricted access. Once back at the hospital, we collected additional water and last-minute snack purchases that the GME administration had delivered to our work rooms.

Wednesday night

Wednesday night was nerve-racking as we watched weather broadcasts in our work room. We huddled in front of the TV, switching between the national and local weather forecasts, as the storm moved closer and closer. We stayed together most of the night, talking to each other and playing video games to keep our spirits up. The hospital food service was in normal operation, so we did not have to dive into our snack stash. It was mostly uneventful in the hospital, even after the hurricane first made landfall. However, I noted the meteorologists reporting from areas on the hurricane's path were moving closer and closer to our town.

Thursday morning

Our residents rounded with the attending physicians who were able to make it in safely as I set up a communications center for updates. Due to the wind and rain damage in the surrounding area, cell towers were not working well, making communication outside the hospital challenging. Using Facebook, WhatsApp, email, and my personal cell phone, I continued to reach out to those sheltering at home to make sure all our residents were making it through the storm safely. I sent the same messages across those four channels because I was unsure what our residents had access to and what they were going through. I was encouraged when colleagues responded, some from home, others from evacuation sites.

The hurricane passed, but there were major concerns about a potential storm surge that might follow. There were rumors that hospital administration had decided that the emergency was over, and Friday would be "business as usual." That did not sit well with me for a few reasons. First, I had heard back from less than 50% of the academic faculty and residents I reached out to, including GME administrators. Second, I was concerned about the impending storm surge, which was projected to peak in a few hours. I spoke with my residents who were already at the hospital. Although they were anxious to check on the status of their own homes, they agreed to stay overnight again. One resident stayed even though he had a fellowship interview the next day, which he would have to do from the hospital after two straight nights in-house. Third, I thought about the duty we had for the patients already under our care and was concerned about a coverage gap if I relieved my current team only to find that residents at home were not able to make it in. Time was of the essence, so in the interest of safety, I made an executive decision to continue running our volunteer crew for an additional night.

Thursday afternoon

When the storm surge came, we weren't fully prepared. The water began to rise and flooded the first-floor parking garage. Word from staff about the garage flooding spread through the hospital. The residents and I walked toward the garage to get a view. There was panic as those who had parked on the first floor rushed to move their vehicles to higher ground. We watched in awe as the storm surge filled the streets with multiple feet of water. Our call rooms and workrooms had windows on the fourth floor, a luxury for residents on a normal day, but could become dangerous in the midst of the storm as the glass could shatter with the strong winds. Water and wind moved boats and cars through the streets like a river. The strong winds destroyed transformers nearby. We resorted to generator power, which further decreased the available space for staff as our GME offices were located outside of the generator. We moved an attending and some of our ICU residents into our workrooms and call rooms due to areas that lost power.

Thursday night

Due to the storm surge, a couple more of our fellow residents stayed over, and we made do with placing air mattresses in our workrooms. In addition, our academic attending lost power in her office, and we offered up one of our call beds in the hospital. Our volunteers banded together and remained positive, despite the cramped space and the concerns about our colleagues and our homes. It was a high-stress environment, and we bonded by spending the night talking to one another on a personal level. We don't always see the human side of each other during normal workdays, so this opportunity was special. I will forever remember one volunteer senior resident. He built a fort on his dining room table around his dog and simply hoped the dog would make it through the storm okay so he could stay at the hospital to take care of his patients. When the storm surge came, the senior resident knew his home was flooded. Attempts to reach his home were futile, as co-residents and their families with trucks were still no match for the depths of the floodwaters. He could do nothing but get through the night, hoping for the best and expecting the worst. The next day, one of my fellow chief residents was able to ride to the senior resident's house. By some miracle, he heard barking when he pulled up to the house. The senior resident was able to get home post-rounds to mend his home and retrieve his dog.

Friday morning

By early morning, the surge had subsided, and my residents checked on their patients. I was concerned that our academic attendings would not be able to get to the hospital. Despite the storm debris and lack of power at their own homes, they arrived at the hospital. A few of our academic attendings were recent graduates of our program and expressed that if they were still residents, they would have volunteered to stay overnight because "that is what we do." They were motivated by the current residents who had volunteered and felt a sense of duty to do the same. It was a relief to see them, and they were welcomed.

Now it was time to organize relief coverage for my team. Using multiple communication channels, we organized a reprieve for those who had spent more than 48 hours in the hospital. I was happy to see people who wanted to come back to work and help, even those who suffered residential damage. I was also thankful for the many interns who wanted to come in. We were fully staffed by Monday, including in our clinic.

Supporting each other in the aftermath of the storm

Those residents who lost their homes stayed with other residents, and a co-chief started a GoFundMe to support the residents with the greatest needs. Even though the hospital offered some support, such as providing gas for staff to make it to their shifts, we wanted to take care of our own. These random acts of kindness among our residency program are why I continue to want to be a part of GME.

I was truly amazed at the selflessness of my colleagues and residents. It didn't matter whether their homes were destroyed, if they were uninhabitable, if they were without power or flooded—everyone wanted to come back to work and help patients and each other.

Looking back, I think that dedication to our patients and to one another is what allowed us to successfully prepare for, staff, and make it through such a challenging time. Preparing for an emergency or natural disaster and then actually going through one can be very different. Working through Hurricane Ian was trying for our residents and chiefs, not just physically, but mentally, as well. Setting fear aside to put our patients first has become second nature for all of us; however, being supportive of each other and banding together when it really matters is what makes us a successful team and a successful program.

NAVIGATING THE PANDEMIC AS A RESIDENT AND A CHIEF RESIDENT

Kaitlin Kyi, MD

University of Rochester School of Medicine and Dentistry

Dr. Kyi, now a hematology/oncology fellow, describes being a senior resident as the COVID-19 pandemic began and becoming a chief resident the following year.

When I was first asked to be chief in the winter of 2019, I imagined the academic year of 2020-2021 would be a time of incredible growth, which turned out to be an understatement. I had not imagined performing chiefly duties while facing a pandemic with an already emotionally depleted group of residents.

I was a "COVID chief" from June 2020 to June 2021. It is still difficult to think about that year, even as I am supremely grateful for its many hard lessons. My co-chiefs and I went into the year fully knowing that service demands might escalate at any time with a secondary wave of COVID-19.

We had finished our last year of residency in the midst of the first wave of COVID-19. Many of us swapped out elective rotations for ICU and inpatient rotations—the "senioritis" of third year never having an opportunity to truly hit us. One rotation—ironically a pulmonary elective—was replaced with a rotation in our COVID intensive care units. While I learned a tremendous amount about proning and ventilation, I recall thinking this was not quite what I had "signed up for." Though the lessons were not what I expected, I would not change a thing.

We had to limit the number of healthcare workers providing hands-on care for COVID-positive patients to prevent spread. I was often the lone provider communicating with family and patients. I remember holding up an iPad for six to eight family members as they said their final goodbyes to their father via video conference. It would be the last time they spoke with him before he was compassionately extubated. "We love you, Dad," they told him over and over again. "We're with you." Their father could not respond; he was sedated and intubated. They were crying, and only because I was safely hidden behind the screen of the tablet, I let myself soundlessly cry, too.

The unique opportunity to provide care in a time of great need unified us as a class. We were tired, we were saddened, but there was an overwhelming sense of duty to rise to the occasion for each other and for our patients. At the time of our class's graduation celebration in June 2020, COVID cases were peaking. Some of us showed up in N95s and scrubs, having just finished shifts. We said our goodbyes to each other as a class, not entirely knowing what the future held.

As we entered our chief year, there was a lull in cases, and we attempted to navigate back to normalcy. Much of this was halted by the ongoing threat of COVID cases spiking in our community and residency colleagues, but we began to reintroduce in-person learning and gatherings, all of which had been put indefinitely on hold. While we had attempted Zoom-based gatherings, there was no surrogate for face-to-face interactions. There was a raucous giddiness to our residents when they were allowed to congregate in conference rooms once more.

Even while we watched the numbers drop, we were ever mindful of summer turning into fall—which is to say, we were constantly tabulating cases and preparing for the "second wave." Even now, I still have a running list in my electronic medical record of COVID-positive patients in our ED and inpatient units—a reminder of how we were constantly assessing and preparing to recalibrate.

As we planned for the fall/winter months, we allotted an increased number of residents for ICU rotations, anticipating an increasing number of patients. But even this careful allotment wasn't enough. By November, the entire hospital system was overtaxed with entire units full of COVID patients. Our hospital medicine and ICU leadership reached out to see if we could reassign more residents to these units. After days of intensive planning, we were able to reallocate residents from our community hospital to our university hospital with the generous help of our family medicine residents who increased inpatient coverage at our community hospital. With their help, we were able to create five additional hospital medicine teams. At every step of this process, we communicated with leadership and residents through both email and online conferences to discuss concerns. There was a sense of urgency in these meetings; all of us were still tired. But there was a sense of a higher obligation to each other and our patients.

We pulled many residents from elective rotations. I can't entirely romanticize these circumstances; a few residents were very frustrated with the continued loss of normalcy. Many of these electives were important, integral to fellowship applications or foundational for learning. I could feel residents avoiding me, as if my friendly greetings were a pretense for yet another sacrifice I would ask them to make. The only thing that mitigated our guilt was our vow to "repay" our residents. With this in mind, we kept a log of the residents who had sacrificed rotations, knowing they would need these learning opportunities once we again returned to whatever was the new normal.

By spring, we began to see a downtick in cases, and we were able to breathe once more. In contrast to the year prior, our third-year residents' graduation was restricted in number, but not one of our residents graduated in an N95 or scrubs.

I said earlier that incredible growth was an understatement for my expectations of chief year. I never could have expected the monumental sacrifice I would have to ask of our residents. Their resilience and strength still humble me. The year taught me how important it is to anticipate, adapt, and communicate as frankly as possible through a crisis.

ACKNOWLEDGMENTS

This book reflects the collective wisdom, work, and support of so many people. I am so sorry if I accidentally left anyone out.

A very special thank you to Susan Davids, who took the reins of the residency program during my sabbatical. I could not have done this without you.

I am also grateful for the patience and grace that my leadership team extended to me while I was working on this project. Thank you, Karen Carlson, Sara Dunbar, Susan Davids, Amy Farkas, Rachel Goodman, Kory Koerner, Morgan Lamberg Hanrahan, Amalia Lyons, Haley Mertens, Brooke Mbow, Michael Putman, Kathy Rafel, Shaina Sekhri, Beth Santiago, and Tracy Stasinopoulos.

Thank you to the residents in my program, past and future. You have made being a program director the most meaningful work I have ever done. You have taught me so much about how to be a better leader. To the chief residents with whom I have worked: Thank you for supporting me as a leader, taking care of the residents in the crises described, and for giving me specific feedback on how to lead with courage and care.

Adina Kalet, thank you for believing that I could do this, and for providing the guidance I needed to get it done.

Thank you to the Medical College of Wisconsin, the Faculty Career Development Committee, and our dean, Joe Kerschner, for the support of my sabbatical. I am also grateful for the support of the Kern Family Foundation, the Department of Internal Medicine, and Department Chair, Roy Silverstein, as well as the Chief of Medicine at the Milwaukee VA Medical

Center, Andreea Anton. So many other faculty members contributed through conversations, ideas, and encouragement: Marty Muntz, Heather Toth, Cassie Ferguson, and Alicia Pilarski to name a few of the most important.

To all the authors who contributed to this book: Thank you for sharing your stories and advice with me and the rest of the world. Since I have not lived through all these crises myself, I could not have written this book without you. I have already learned so much from your wisdom, and I am certain that others will, too.

To Mark Maltarich, PhD, my Chapter 1 and 2 co-author, I am amazed by your deep knowledge of the teamwork literature and so happy that you agreed to work on this project with me. Spending time with you and Kathleen in Columbia established the trajectory for this book.

I am so grateful for all who provided a sanctuary for me to write the book. Thank you to my aunt Sally Duncan McCaskey and Clay McCaskey who hosted me in Hilton Head while I drafted the most difficult chapter in the book. To my sister, Wendy Franzen, thank you for providing so many days and nights of quiet refuge away from the bustle of my house. It is so easy to reflect and write in your peaceful garden. Thank you, Joan Neuner, for our writing retreat at your home by Lake Michigan to kick off the start of the spring sabbatical.

I am lucky to have a friend, Liam Callanan, who is a fiction writer. Thank you for having coffee with me and showing me how to make the dry "cases" in these pages become relatable "stories."

I have so many colleagues, friends, and a daughter (!) who reviewed drafts of chapters for me. I appreciate the insight and edits that you provided: Bruce Campbell, Lorna Dilley, Sarah Dotters-Katz, Kathleen Finn, Michael Frank, Lily Littrell, Jeff Jackson, Lindsey Loveland Baptist, Joan Neuner, Elise Papke, Marilyn Schapira, Ralph Schapira, Jennifer Schmidt, Rachel Simmons, and Kathryn West. Three people reviewed the *entire* draft and gave me very helpful constructive feedback. Darcy Reed, Paula M. Termuhlen, and Abigail Ford Winkel, thank you for the time you spent making this book so much better.

Thank you to David Cipriano, PhD, for providing important content in the Campus Crisis chapter and for talking me through the crises I have faced as a program director.

Nancy Duran, you are an extraordinary risk manager for the MCW graduate medical education office. There is literally not a single crisis that I have navigated without you. Thank you for your relentless composure and the personal support you have given me over the years.

Karen Herzog, you are a fantastic editor. I was so nervous to hand this off to someone, but your care of the words and messages in these chapters was evident from the start. Thank you for making this book shine.

To my exercise group, thank you for keeping me moving forward, literally, especially my carpool buddies Kim Khan and Lorna Dilley. To my book club, thank you for promising to have this book be one of our selections. To the rest of my friend group, you have inspired me and helped me find balance with humor and love during the crises described herein, so thank you.

To my family . . . Lily, thank you for sharing your art with the world through the book and its cover. I love the times that we have sat together doing art on the back porch and talking about our worlds. Jay, you have shown me that our imperfections make our progress even more meaningful than if we were always perfect. Luke, thank you for our evening ritual of sharing what we are grateful for. I love that you call me when I am not at home to make sure that we do it every night. Jack, thank you for literally everything, and for already introducing me as "Kathlyn Fletcher, author." Jane, Carl, Oma, Sam, Liz, Haley, Fabi, Evy, Franzi, Elly, Ronja, and the rest of our family, you are the support system that makes all our family achievements possible.

Dad, I hope that you can see some of the pragmatic advice you have given me over the years in these pages. I am grateful for your love and belief in me.

Mom, I think about you every day . . . your love, grace, and perseverance. I think that you would be proud of this work. I hope so.

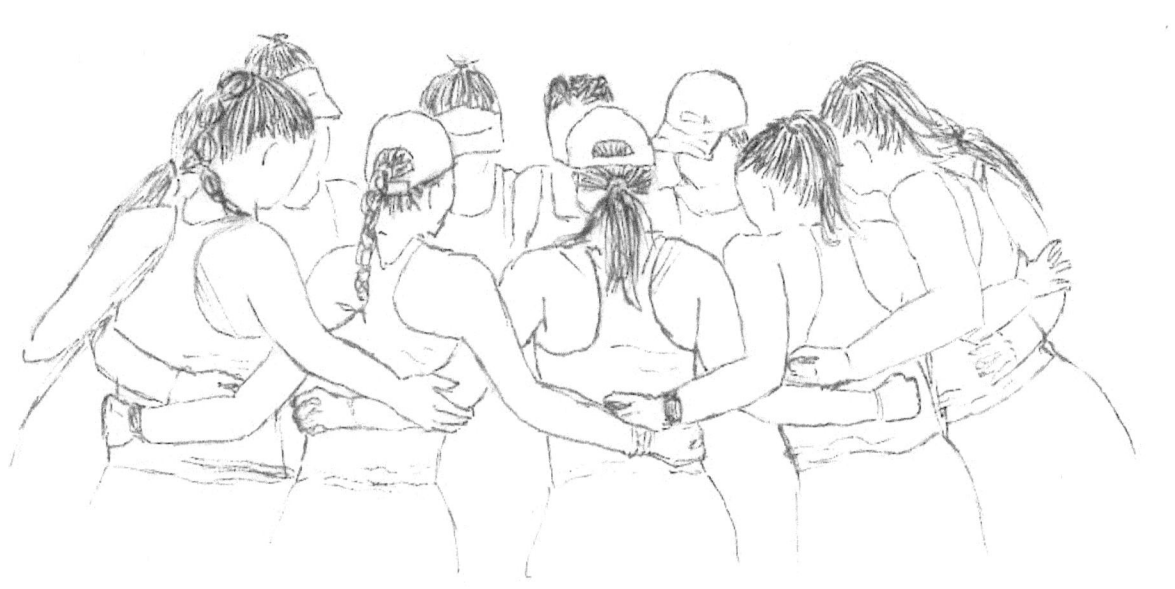

www.ingramcontent.com/pod-product-compliance
Lightning Source LLC
Chambersburg PA
CBHW081330230426
43667CB00018B/2887